An Innocent Baby

ALSO BY CATHY GLASS

FOSTERING MEMOIRS

Cut
The Silent Cry
Daddy's Little Princess
Nobody's Son
Cruel to be Kind
The Night the Angels Came
A Long Way from Home
A Baby's Cry
The Saddest Girl in the World
Please Don't Take My Baby
Will You Love Me?
I Miss Mummy
Saving Danny
Girl Alone
Where Has Mummy Gone?
Damaged
Hidden
Mummy Told Me Not to Tell
Another Forgotten Child
The Child Bride
Can I Let You Go?
Finding Stevie
Innocent
Too Scared to Tell
A Terrible Secret
A Life Lost

INSPIRED BY EXPERIENCE

The Girl in the Mirror
My Dad's a Policeman
Run, Mummy, Run

SHARING HER EXPERTISE

Happy Kids
Happy Adults
Happy Mealtimes for Kids
About Writing and How to
Publish

WRITING AS LISA STONE

The Darkness Within
Stalker
The Doctor
Taken
The Cottage

THE MILLION COPY BESTSELLING AUTHOR

CATHY GLASS

An Innocent Baby

Why would anyone abandon
little Darcy-May?

Certain details in this story, including names, places and dates, have been changed to protect the family's privacy.

HarperElement
An imprint of HarperCollins*Publishers*
1 London Bridge Street
London SE1 9GF

www.harpercollins.co.uk

HarperCollins*Publishers*
1st Floor, Watermarque Building, Ringsend Road
Dublin 4, Ireland

First published by HarperElement 2021

3 5 7 9 10 8 6 4

A catalogue record of this book is
available from the British Library

ISBN 978-0-00-846648-0

Printed and bound in the UK using 100%
renewable electricity at CPI Group (UK) Ltd

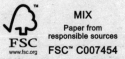

MIX
Paper from
responsible sources
FSC™ C007454

This book is produced from independently certified FSC™ paper
to ensure responsible forest management.

For more information visit: www.harpercollins.co.uk/green

ACKNOWLEDGEMENTS

A big thank you to my family; my editors, Kelly and Holly; my literary agent, Andrew; my UK publisher HarperCollins; and my overseas publishers, who are now too numerous to list by name. Last, but definitely not least, a big thank you to my readers for your unfailing support and kind words. They are much appreciated.

To my darling mother.
Forever in our hearts.

AUTHOR'S NOTE

As a foster carer I can usually find some sympathy for parents whose children have been taken into care, as so often they've struggled with life's challenges themselves. But I had no sympathy whatsoever for Haylea's father, who was evil beyond words. I struggled to write this book at times, but Haylea's story needed to be told to raise awareness and hopefully save others.

CHAPTER ONE

ADRIAN'S WISH IS GRANTED

After my mother died I took three months off from fostering. As well as grieving for her, there was a lot to do: informing friends and the wider family of her passing, arranging the funeral, and then clearing out and selling her home. That final visit to her house was heart-wrenching. It was where I had grown up and where she had lived for most of her married life. It contained so many memories. As I closed the front door for the last time I felt a devastating finality. My children felt it too. That part of our lives had now gone for good. No more visits to Nana and all that encompassed. Her welcoming hugs, kisses and smiles. Her endless patience, empathy, love and kindness. Her cups of tea and freshly baked cakes, and the way she would wave us off at the door as we left.

Mum had always welcomed the children I fostered as one of the family, and in twenty-five years of fostering that was a lot of children. Many of them were still in touch with me and when I told them of Nana's passing they were greatly saddened, but able to recount lots of happy memories of when they'd seen her at her house or mine. I was on the phone for hours listening to and sharing in their recollections, and their words really helped. Mum was treasured by them as she was by us and so many of my readers. Thank you for all your kind messages. Quite a few of those I'd fostered came to Mum's funeral. The church was packed.

I'd arranged a buffet lunch for the wake, which gave us a chance to catch up and share in the joy of having known Mum. Many remembered my father too. It was wonderful to know that my parents lived on in the hearts of so many. My family and I consoled ourselves that after a long and happy life Mum was at rest with my father.

Towards the end of March I told Joy, my supervising social worker (SSW), that I felt ready to foster again. All carers in the UK have an SSW to monitor and support their fostering, and referrals for children needing a foster home are usually made through them. I'd previously discussed with Joy the possibility of fostering a young child or baby. Adrian, my adult son, was moving out in June to marry his long-term girlfriend and fiancée, Kirsty, and he was worried that without him I might be in danger if an angry teenager or older child kicked off. I thought he was worrying unnecessarily and pointed out that carers can't pick and choose, and an angry child needs a loving home just as any child does, which Adrian knew. But I'd agreed to mention it to Joy.

The day after I'd said I was able to foster again Joy phoned me with a referral.

'Adrian's wish has been granted,' she began lightly. 'There's a newborn in the city hospital, a little girl, two days old.' Immediately I felt my eyes fill.

'At present she is being cared for by the nurses,' Joy continued. 'But she's ready to go now they are satisfied she's feeding. She's coming straight into foster care. Can you take her?'

'Yes,' I said, and my heart clenched. A little baby separated from her mother at birth. Why? I wondered. Would they ever see each other again?

'She weighs six pounds,' Joy continued. 'There is no sign of drug dependency.'

'Good.' If the mother is an addict the baby is often born drug-dependent and needs a programme to wean them off it. They can be in agony as they suffer withdrawal.

'Her mother has called the baby Darcy-May, but there won't be any contact.'

'None at all?' I asked in dismay.

'No. I understand the baby will go for adoption. Their social worker will have more details when she calls you. They really need to move the baby today, but I said you would need time to prepare as it's some years since you fostered a baby.'

'Yes, that's right.'

'So, I can tell the social worker you will have Darcy-May tomorrow?'

'Yes. I expect they'll want me to collect her from the hospital – I think that's what happened the last time I fostered a baby. I'll need to get the car seat down from the loft,' I said, thinking aloud.

'Yes, but you won't need the car seat tomorrow,' Joy said. 'Darcy-May will be brought to you. The family are known to the police and they want to make sure she's not followed to your house. They must never find out where the baby is.'

And that was the first inkling I had of the horror story that lay ahead.

3

CHAPTER TWO

DARCY-MAY ARRIVES

Having agreed to foster Darcy-May, I spent the rest of the day getting ready for her arrival. Straight after Joy's phone call I dashed into town and bought bottles, nappies, formula, creams, wipes and so on, together with a new mattress for the cot. The cot, car seat, Moses basket and stroller were stored in the loft, but I'd thrown out the mattress after the last baby I'd fostered.

Just as I'd finished shopping and was loading the bags into the car, Joy phoned again, and for one moment I thought she was going to tell me it was all off and that Darcy-May wouldn't be coming to me after all. Such last-minute changes in fostering can and do happen. However, she said she'd spoken to Shari, the social worker responsible for Darcy-May and her mother (who I now learnt was called Haylea), and could confirm that Shari would bring the baby to me the following morning.

'Shari is going to try to phone you later,' Joy said. 'But she's in court all day. If she doesn't get the chance, she said she'll see you tomorrow.'

'OK. Do you know what time she'll be arriving?' I asked.

'No. She's not sure. She said as early as she could.'

I drove home, unpacked and prepared for the following day as best I could. I would wait until Adrian, twenty-eight, or my daughter Paula, twenty-four, returned home from work to help me get the items down from the loft. In the meantime I telephoned my other daughter, Lucy, aged twenty-six. She was now living with her partner, Darren, and their baby Emma – my first grandchild, who was nearly eight months old. Lucy was delighted when I told her I would be fostering a newborn, although, like me, she was sad the baby couldn't stay with her mother.

'We can go for walks in the park together, Mum,' she said. 'And I've got some first-size baby clothes you can have. They've hardly been used. But why isn't the mother keeping her baby?' she asked, concerned.

'I don't know yet. I should find out more when the social worker phones later, or tomorrow when she brings the baby. I've been told very little.'

'That seems a bit strange for a planned move,' Lucy said.

'Yes.'

Lucy knew how the social services worked from being in care herself. She'd come to me as a foster child and I'd subsequently adopted her. She couldn't have been more loved and cherished if she'd been born to me. I tell Lucy's story in *Will You Love Me?*

'The baby is called Darcy-May,' I added.

'That's a nice name.'

'Yes, it is.'

I didn't tell Lucy that the baby's family was known to the police. She didn't need to know that, and she'd worry. I said only that the family wouldn't know where Darcy-May was, which wasn't so unusual. If a parent puts a child into care voluntarily and is working with the social services and has regular contact with the child with a view to them going home, they are likely to be told where the child is. But if the child is at risk of harm from the parents then this information is withheld, although sometimes it's accidentally divulged.

When Adrian and Paula arrived home from work I told them the same as I'd told Lucy. They were both pleased I would be fostering a baby but expressed the same sadness as Lucy had – that the mother wasn't able to keep her child. I couldn't tell them any more, as I hadn't heard from the social worker. I pass on information to my family about the child we are fostering on a need-to-know basis.

After dinner they helped me get the equipment down from the loft. We set the Moses basket on its stand in my bedroom, then assembled the cot beside it. I'd use the Moses basket for the first few weeks and, following current guidelines, Darcy-May would sleep in my bedroom for at least six months. Longer if there were any concerns about her health. Assuming she was still with us, she'd then sleep in the cot in a room of her own.

I was as prepared as I could be and, thanking Adrian and Paula for their help, I sat in the living room with a mug of tea where our cat, Sammy, was curled up in his usual chair. My thoughts went to Darcy-May and her mother, Haylea, of whom I knew nothing. There are nearly two thousand infants taken into care in the UK each year and each has their own sorry story. Some of the infants can return to their mothers, but many have to be found new homes, either with a suitable relative or through adoption. Like many foster carers, I've always found fostering a baby bittersweet. They give us so much joy, but we are acutely aware that a mother is without her baby, and then at some point we have to say goodbye, which is very painful.

It was at moments like this, when I felt a little down-hearted and reflective, that I would have telephoned my dear mother for a chat. A few reassuring words from her always helped, but of course that was no longer possible. Fortunately, Adrian appeared with a smile.

'Kirsty's mother wants you to check the seating plan for the wedding reception again,' he said with a little sigh. 'She's emailed a copy to you. I'm sure it's fine, but can you let her know?'

'Yes, of course, love. I'll have a look at it now.' It was only three months to the wedding and Kirsty's mother, Andrea, was doing a fantastic job of organizing everything and everyone.

'Thanks, I'll be relieved when it's all over,' he said.

'Don't worry. It will be fine.'

I checked the seating plan on my tablet and emailed Kirsty's mother to say it was looking good. I then made some notes for an article I'd been asked to write. Since I'd been publishing my fostering memoirs, I'd also been asked to write articles about raising children based on my years of fostering experience. Before going to bed I made sure everything I needed for making up baby feeds was to hand in the kitchen: the bottles, sterilizing unit, formula and so forth. I knew from experience that a hungry baby doesn't like to be kept waiting.

* * *

I'm an early riser – a habit from years of looking after children, as I like to be showered and dressed before the child in order to keep on top of the day. As it turned out it was just as well I was up at my usual time for, soon after I had seen Adrian and Paula off to work, the front doorbell rang. It was nearly 8.30 a.m. so I assumed it was a parcel or a letter that required a signature. But as I opened the door I was surprised to see a police officer with a woman beside him, cradling a bundle swaddled in white.

'Cathy Glass?' she asked.

'Yes. Hello. Come in,' I flustered.

'I'm Shari.' Then, turning to the officer, she said, 'You can go now. Thank you for your help. I'll call a cab when I'm ready to leave.'

The officer handed me the briefcase he was carrying for Shari and returned down the path to the police car parked outside. I closed the front door and looked at the tiny baby.

'Oh my,' I swooned. 'She's so cute.' Her little face was just visible over the blanket and under the white hat. Her eyes were tightly closed.

'She's lost a little of her birth weight as most babies do,' Shari said. 'But the nurse said she should soon make it up. She's been feeding well. I've got her hospital notes in my briefcase. Which room are we in?'

'This way,' I said. Carrying Shari's briefcase, I led the way down the hall to our living room. 'Would you like a coffee?' I asked her.

'Yes, please. Milk, no sugar.'

I made Shari a coffee and placed it on the occasional table in the living room within her reach. She had laid Darcy-May on the sofa beside her.

'I'll fetch the Moses basket so we can put her in that,' I suggested. I went upstairs and brought down the basket and stand, then set it up in the living room. Shari carefully lowered Darcy-May into the Moses basket, removing the blanket she'd been wrapped in. I'd already put bedding in the Moses basket and I tucked her in. Darcy-May screwed up her nose but remained asleep.

'When was she last fed?' I asked, as Shari sat down.

'Just before I left the hospital.'

'I'll make up some bottles of formula later. I was going to do it before you came.' I sat in the armchair close to the Moses basket.

'I've got a bottle of formula you can have. The hospital gave it to me.' She took it from her briefcase and placed it on the coffee table. 'And here are the placement forms,' she added, setting those beside the bottle. I would read them later. She drank some of her coffee and then said, 'We wanted to move Darcy-May early before Haylea's father got wind of it. He's been turning up regularly at the hospital, creating a fuss and threatening the staff. He doesn't want the baby taken into care. He's very rude and aggressive. We weren't followed here. The police were very good. I've given the hospital your contact details and a midwife will be in touch.' She paused to drink her coffee.

'Where does the family live?' I asked.

She named a neighbouring town. 'You are unlikely to bump into them here, but I wouldn't go shopping there. Haylea is in a residential children's home. She doesn't want to go home.'

'I see. How old is she then?' I asked

'Fourteen. Nearly fifteen.'

'Dear me. That is young to have a baby. And the baby's father?'

'We don't know. Haylea is refusing to give any details, probably because she knows he would be in trouble.' It's illegal in the UK to have penetrative sex with a person under the age of sixteen. 'Haylea didn't have any antenatal care,' Shari said. 'She just turned up at the hospital complaining of stomach cramps. She says she didn't know she was pregnant.'

'Good grief. Is that possible?'

'Not sure. It's what Haylea is saying, and when we spoke to her father he told us to mind our own fucking business.'

'Charming.'

'Haylea doesn't want anything to do with the baby, so it will go straight for adoption. Which reminds me,' she said, 'I will need to register the birth.' She made a note.

'Didn't anyone else notice she was pregnant?' I asked. 'Her school? Friends? Others in her family?'

'She hasn't been going to school. I don't know about friends. As far as we can see there is no one else living permanently at home, apart from her father. Social services were involved some years ago soon after the mother left,' Shari continued. 'The father had a new part-ner and it was decided they were doing a reasonable job of looking after Haylea. It now seems the woman wasn't there for long and left soon after our visit. Haylea has three older siblings. Two brothers, one who is in prison and we are not sure where the other one is. Her older sister ran away from home soon after the mother left.'

'So Haylea has had very little in the way of support?' I said.

Shari nodded. 'The father has a history of causing fights and other criminal activity. He says he wants Haylea and the baby home, but that's not going to happen. It's no place for a baby and Haylea doesn't want any more to do with him. If he should show up here, call the police.'

'I will, but that's not likely, is it?' I asked, even more concerned.

'Hopefully not. But it wouldn't do any harm to be cautious.' Which did nothing to help my unease. 'To be honest, the sooner that poor baby is settled with adoptive parents and able to start her new life, the better.'

I agreed. Without good family support, Haylea wouldn't be able to bring up the baby. She was only a child herself. Also, for whatever reason, she had decided she didn't want anything to do with it.

Shari checked I had everything I needed for fostering a baby and asked me to sign the placement agreement, which forms the contract the carer has with the local authority to foster the child. She called a cab and while she waited for it to arrive she looked around the house, as social workers are expected to do at each visit.

Having seen Shari out, I checked on Darcy-May, who was still asleep, so I took the opportunity to make up bottles of formula, following the instructions on the packet. I texted my family's WhatsApp group to tell them that Darcy-May had arrived and was looking forward to meeting them soon, then I sat beside the Moses basket, gazing at her. As I looked I saw her bottom lip start to move, a sign she could be hungry. I went to fetch one of the bottles of formula and checked the temperature of the milk. Just in time. As I returned to the living room her little face screwed up and her mouth opened as she began to cry; that piercing newborn baby hunger scream that can't be ignored.

'There, there,' I soothed, and picked her up.

I sat in the armchair with her cradled close to my chest and offered the bottle. There was a little hesitation, another cry, and then she latched onto the teat. I was relieved. Sometimes newborn babies take a while to realize that a teat means food.

As I sat there watching Darcy-May feed I thought how much my dear mother would have enjoyed me fostering a baby, just as the rest of my family would. But what of Haylea? I wondered. Where was she right now? What was she doing, thinking and feeling? As she was a minor, the social services had a duty to look after her. Perhaps in time she would be able to start a new life, just as her daughter would be doing. Return to school, get some qualifications, a job and eventually, hopefully, form a loving relationship. In years to come when Darcy-May was an adult she could, if she wished, find her birth mother, assuming Haylea agreed. I love happy endings and as I sat there gazing adoringly at Darcy-May I pictured her as a young woman reunited with her birth mother while her adoptive parents looked on, smiling.

I was soon jolted from my thoughts. Darcy-May finished feeding and a powerful smell rose from her nappy.

'Time to change you,' I said. I stood and carefully carried her upstairs to my bedroom where I was keeping the nappies, wipes and creams.

I didn't have a changing station as I rarely fostered babies, but I'd bought a changing mat while I'd been shopping. I placed that on my bed, with the nappies, wipes and other items I needed within reach. Darcy-May was content as I laid her down but like many babies didn't like the feel of having her nappy changed. As soon as I took off the old one she began to cry very loudly.

'Sshh, it's OK,' I said, trying to comfort her as I cleaned her. She cried all the more.

Then the house phone began to ring, as it always seems to at such moments. I ignored it for as long as I could, but the ringing seemed to be upsetting Darcy-May even more, so with the old nappy off and the new ready to put on, I reached out and picked up the extension. 'Hello?' I asked as Darcy-May hollered in the background.

'I guess this isn't a good time,' Joy said.

'I'm just changing her. I'll phone you once she's settled.'

Returning the receiver to its cradle, I finished changing Darcy-May and then carried her downstairs. Comfortable again, she was soon asleep so I placed her in the Moses basket, then returned Joy's call. She was checking that all was well and said she would visit tomorrow. Supervising social workers, like the child's social workers, are expected to visit the foster carer regularly.

The rest of the day passed happily with Darcy-May sleeping between feeds, which allowed me the chance to get on with other jobs, including housework. So when Adrian and Paula arrived home from work at six o'clock it was to a calm and well-ordered house. I felt pleased with myself. Dinner was ready and Darcy-May, having just had another bottle, was fast asleep in the Moses basket. It didn't last long.

CHAPTER THREE

VISITORS

Almost the second Adrian, Paula and I had finished dinner Darcy-May began crying, and from then on we had a very unsettled evening. Perhaps it was colic – although I had winded her – or maybe the formula was different to the one she was used to or she was reacting to the change in surroundings. I didn't know.

'Maybe she's hungry,' Paula suggested as I picked her up yet again.

'She could be, although she had a bottle half an hour ago.'

'Shall I get another one so you can try?' Paula offered.

'Yes, please, love, but warm it first.'

Paula disappeared into the kitchen while Adrian stood watching me rocking Darcy-May.

'For someone so small, she can make a lot of noise,' he remarked.

I smiled. 'I seem to remember you had a good pair of lungs too.' I sat on the sofa and gently rubbed her back. Adrian was still watching me. 'Would you like a go?' I asked.

'Sure.'

Adrian sat beside me and I carefully transferred Darcy-May into his arms. He is sturdily built and over six feet tall; Darcy-May seemed even smaller now lying in the crook of his arm. But Adrian is a gentle giant and as he cooed, rocked and tried to calm her I was very touched. I knew he would make a great father if he and Kirsty had children.

Darcy-May stopped crying, but only briefly. Paula returned with the bottle and Adrian tried her with it, but she wasn't interested and grew more upset. There's nothing quite like a crying baby to make you feel helpless.

'What does she want?' Adrian asked.

'Not sure,' I replied. 'Sometimes babies cry for no obvious reason.'

I offered her the bottle, but she didn't want to know. I then walked around the room with her in my arms until she fell asleep. But the moment I put her in the Moses basket she started crying again.

'I'll see to the dishes, Mum,' Adrian offered.

'Thanks, love.'

Paula stayed with me as I tried to comfort Darcy-May and eventually she was ready for another feed and took the formula milk. I winded her and put her in the Moses basket, where she slept for an hour before she woke again, crying. And so it continued throughout the evening. If she'd had a temperature or a rash or any other sign she might be unwell, I would have sought medical help. I seemed to remember that when Paula had been a baby she'd become fractious in the evenings for the first few weeks for no apparent reason.

In the middle of all of this Lucy telephoned and spoke to Adrian, who said I was seeing to Darcy-May. She told him she'd see me tomorrow and sent her love.

At nine o'clock I decided to try to settle Darcy-May in my bedroom, ready for the night. I needed to try to establish a routine of sorts. Adrian took the Moses basket and stand upstairs and set it up in my bedroom as Paula helped me give Darcy-May a sponge bath, which I thought might comfort her. I used the sink in the bathroom, as she was so small and I knew I should keep the umbilical cord stub dry. Darcy-May cried as we removed her clothes, but once seated in the warm water she relaxed. Paula supported her back and head as I sponged the warm water over her. Using cotton wool, I gently cleaned around the umbilical cord stub. It would drop off in about one to two weeks. Once Darcy-May was bathed, Paula held out the large fluffy towel I'd bought especially for her and I lifted her into it.

'She smells so nice,' Paula said, holding her close. 'Especially her hair.'

'Yes, she does. I love that warm, cosy baby smell.' I stroked her cheek and she seemed to smile, although it was probably wind.

Paula carried her, wrapped in the towel, into my bedroom where I closed the curtains and switched on the dimmer light. Together we put a new nappy on Darcy-May and then her vest and sleepsuit.

'Night, night,' Paula said, kissing her. 'I'll be in my room if you need me, Mum.'

'Thanks for your help.'

I sat on my bed and with the light down low gave Darcy-May a bottle, which I hoped would see her off to sleep for a few hours at least. I tucked her into the Moses basket and, switching on the baby monitor, came out, quietly closing the door. Downstairs I made myself a mug of tea and then sat in the living room with the microphone from the monitor beside me and opened my laptop. I should start my log notes for Darcy-May while I had the chance. Foster carers in the UK are required to keep a record of the child or children they are looking after. This includes appointments and details of the child's health and wellbeing. As well as charting their progress, it can act as an aide-mémoire if necessary. These notes, like most other records, are now stored digitally. I logged into the Local Authority portal and began.

I could hear Darcy-May murmuring and snuffling through the monitor, then there was a little grizzle. I stopped typing and waited. It went quiet and stayed quiet, so I went upstairs to check on her. She was fast asleep. I returned downstairs but checked on her every time the monitor went quiet. Yes, I was being overly cautious, but it's a huge responsibility, caring for a baby, especially when it's not your own.

Sammy, our cat, finally appeared. He'd kept well away from Darcy-May and seemed scared of her, which was good in a way. I knew we had to be vigilant with Sammy and the baby. If a cat jumps into a baby's crib and snuggles up close, they can suffocate the baby. Sammy wasn't allowed upstairs, but I'd closed my bedroom door anyway, and I would be keeping a close eye on him during the day as well. The longer he remained wary of her, the better.

I stayed up until Darcy-May woke for her next feed and then, having changed her, went to bed myself. It was just after midnight, but I didn't sleep. I lay in the dark, listening to the sounds coming from the Moses basket. I'd forgotten how noisy babies could be when asleep and I wasn't used to having someone else in my bedroom. I'd been divorced for many years. Every grunt, snuffle, groan and coo had me wide awake. At one point it sounded as though she was chuckling and I smiled too.

Darcy-May woke every two to three hours for a feed during the night and by the morning I felt as though I hadn't had any sleep at all. But I didn't mind. Far worse than a baby crying is one that doesn't cry at all. Some infants who are brought into care have been so badly neglected that they've learnt not to cry, as their needs are never met. They just lie silent in their cots, staring up, withdrawn and unresponsive. It's heart-breaking and takes many months of loving care, interaction and stimulation from the foster carer before they begin to respond and eventually thrive.

I could catch up on my sleep during the day while Darcy slept, I thought, as I got up at 6 a.m. to feed her again. It wasn't as though I had another child to look after, and with no contact I would be having an easy time of it. If the care plan is that the baby will return to the mother, then contact is usually every day. Although this is essential to establish and maintain a bond between the mother and her child, it can be very time-consuming and disruptive for the carer and their family.

I fed and changed Darcy-May while still in my nightwear and then, as she slept again, I showered and dressed. Downstairs I fed Sammy, let him out for a run and then made up more bottles of formula, which I put in the fridge. Adrian and Paula were up at 7 a.m. as they had to leave at around 8.15 to go to work. Neither of them had heard Darcy-May during the night, probably because I'd answered her calls immediately. Indeed, Adrian assumed she'd slept through!

'That would be very unusual for a newborn,' I said.

Darcy-May woke again just before 9 a.m. and I fed and changed her in my bedroom. Then I took her and the Moses basket downstairs and settled her in the living room. It was a routine that would see me through the next few weeks.

While she slept I made myself another coffee and took the opportunity to read the placement forms Shari had left yesterday. It included the consent form I needed to allow me to seek emergency medical treatment for Darcy-May should it be necessary. But as I flicked through the pages I saw that the boxes which should have contained information were largely blank. Some of this was because that part of the form was only relevant to older children, where details of nursery, school, language, emotional development, interests and any challenging behaviour were noted. What information there was about Darcy-May I already knew. Her date of birth, mother's name and age. But the box for her contact details was blank. Darcy-May's ethnicity was shown as white British; her legal status was that she was the subject of an Interim Care Order, leading to a Full Care Order and adoption. Details of her health included the name of the hospital where she was born, that her birth had been normal, she was healthy and weighed six pounds one ounce. It stated that her mother hadn't received any antenatal care, which again I already knew. The box for dietary requirements said that three-hour feeding had been established with formula baby milk. The page where key workers were listed showed Shari's and her team manager's names and work contact details. Beside contact arrangements for Darcy-May was typed *None*. The box for other significant persons was also blank, although further down it stated that Haylea had been living with her father and had no contact with her mother and siblings. Never before had I seen a placement form so full of blanks. Darcy-May was alone in this world. All she had was us.

I set the form to one side and, deep in thought, finished my coffee. A key went in the front door and Lucy's voice called, 'Hi, Mum, it's me!' Just as she used to when she'd lived here and returned home, only now of course she had my granddaughter with her.

I immediately stood and went into the hall to greet them. 'Hello, love,' I said, hugging and kissing them both. 'How are you?'

'Good. Where is she?' Lucy asked.

'In the living room.'

Everyone loves a new baby, and I had the impression that Lucy had come to see little Darcy-May as much as she'd come to see me. She passed Emma to me and slipped off her shoes. Emma smiled adorably, waved her arms in the air, and with a cry of delight snuggled her face into my cheek. I kissed her and she babbled away as if she was talking. I saw Emma regularly, but even in the space of a few days she seemed to have developed.

We went into the living room where Lucy stood at the Moses basket, gazing down on Darcy-May, while I sat with Emma on my lap. I took some toys from the toy box for her to play with.

'She's gorgeous. Like a little doll,' Lucy said, admiring Darcy-May. 'You forget how tiny they are at this age.' But it wasn't long before Lucy became serious and sad.

'Isn't her mother seeing her at all?' she asked.

'No. She's only fourteen and has made the decision to give her up for adoption. She hasn't anyone at home to support her.'

'Oh dear, how sad. But you do need a lot of support with a baby. I'm twenty-six and have Darren, his family, you, Adrian and Paula. Yet there were still times when I felt I was sinking. It's easier now Emma is sleeping through the night. I feel human again, but those early weeks passed in a blur.'

'You did fine,' I reassured her.

'But to have no one must be dreadful.'

'Yes, I feel sorry for her.'

'Will you meet her mother?' Lucy asked.

'I don't think so.'

'If she saw her baby, she might not be able to give her up,' Lucy said. But Lucy knew as I did that there were other factors involved. If the social services decided that Haylea couldn't provide adequate parenting to raise her baby, then they could place her for adoption without her consent – through a court order.

Emma wanted to be put down on the floor, and I admired her crawling. She'd only recently started crawling, so it was still a little jerky. She scampered a short way and then stopped as if she couldn't believe she was moving. It was comical, but eventually she reached the toy box and began to amuse herself. Lucy and I talked as Emma played. When Darcy-May woke for a feed Lucy wanted to give her the bottle, which was fine until Emma got jealous and grizzled, wanting to be picked up. I tried but she wanted her mother, so we swapped and I took Darcy-May.

Lucy stayed for the rest of the morning and left at 12.30. She was returning home to give Emma some lunch before taking her to a mother-and-baby group in the afternoon. I kissed and hugged them both goodbye at the door and then went into the kitchen to make myself a sandwich lunch. Before I'd taken the first bite the front doorbell rang. It was too early for Joy, my SSW – she wasn't due until three o'clock. Leaving my untouched sandwich, I answered the door. A woman wearing a royal-blue tunic with a shoulder bag and a small case stood there.

'Cathy Glass?' she asked.

'Yes.'

'I'm Arabell Turner. Midwife. I understand you are looking after a baby girl, Darcy-May.'

'Yes, that's correct. Come in. I'm her foster carer.' I'd been expecting the midwife to visit at some point – it's usual when a newborn baby returns home – but I thought she would have phoned first to make an appointment. 'She's in the living room,' I said, and led the way.

'How is she doing?' Arabell asked.

'All right. I'm feeding her on demand about every three hours.'

'Good.' Setting down her case, she looked in the crib. 'What a dear little mite. She seems very content. I'll have to disturb her later to check her over, but I can do the paperwork first.'

She sat in the armchair next to the crib and took a laptop from her shoulder bag. 'We've gone digital,' she said with a sigh. 'But I have the Red Book in my bag for you. That's still physical.'

As she waited for her laptop to load, she took the Red Book from her bag and passed it to me. This is the Personal Child Health Record, or PCHR. It's known as the 'Red Book' simply because the book has a red cover. It contains the baby's details and a record of their growth and development – weight, body measurements, immunizations and so on. I would need to take it to all Darcy-May's medical appointments so it could be updated. Eventually it would go with her to her adoptive parents.

'Did you deliver Darcy-May?' I asked as we waited.

'No, a colleague on the night shift did. By the time I arrived the next morning the mother had gone. I never met her. I was out this way so offered to make this call.' Usually the mother-to-be builds up a relationship with the midwife during her antenatal care, but Haylea hadn't had any antenatal care.

'The mother didn't stay long in hospital,' I said.

'No. Apparently she was eager to leave. There were no complications, so the doctor discharged her. She has an appointment for a postnatal check-up in six weeks' time. Have you met her?'

'No, and I'm not likely to. There is no contact and the baby is going for adoption.'

'Probably for the best, poor little thing,' she said, pulling a sorrowful face. 'I understand the grandfather has been going into the hospital causing trouble. Does he know where the baby is?'

'No.'

'Good. Keep it that way.' She paused and tapped the keypad. 'Here it is. Normally a midwife visits the mother and baby at home for the first few weeks to help with the mother's postpartum care,' she said. 'Then the health visitor takes over. But that doesn't really apply to you as you didn't give birth. So, if you're happy, I will record this visit and then pass to the health visitor for the next one.'

'Yes, that's fine with me.'

She spent a few moments scrolling down and studying the file. 'A lot of this form isn't relevant. It's about the mother, so I'll just put *Not applicable; baby with foster carer*.'

I nodded.

She then asked standard questions about the baby, the formula she was on, how much and how often she was taking her feed, if her nappies were wet – which they were. Dry nappies can be a sign the baby is dehydrated. Did she have a soiled nappy each day? 'Yes,' I replied. Had the umbilical cord fallen off yet? No – although she would check it when she examined the baby. 'Any signs of jaundice?'

'No.'

'She has a good colour,' she said, peering into the Moses basket.

Once she'd finished, she examined Darcy-May, who didn't like being woken and having her clothes taken off. She cried as the midwife examined her, listened to her heart, looked in her eyes and mouth and at the umbilical cord stub. Arabell took portable scales from her case and I gently placed Darcy-May onto the tray. She noted the results.

'There's just the heel-prick test,' she said.

I held Darcy-May and braced myself, as I knew what was coming: her heel would be pricked and a drop of blood taken and tested for several diseases, including cystic fibrosis and sickle-cell disease. She screamed as the needle pricked her skin.

'I am sorry,' Arabell said, and placed the sample in a sealable plastic bag.

Darcy-May wasn't really due for another feed yet, but as she was so upset I took her with me into the kitchen where I quickly warmed a bottle of milk. I returned to the living room where Arabell was putting away her laptop.

'She'll soon calm down,' she said with a professional smile, and headed towards the door. I followed, baby and bottle in hand. 'The health visitor will be in touch,' she said.

'Thank you.'

Having seen her out, I returned to the living room. Darcy-May took some of her bottle and fell asleep, so I laid her in the Moses basket. The room was warm and I was tired from a broken night. I leant my head back and closed my eyes with the intention of just resting for a few minutes. I must have dropped off, for suddenly the front doorbell was ringing. It was three o'clock so it would be Joy. Darcy-May had been startled by the ringing too and began crying loudly. I picked her up and answered the door with a screaming baby in my arms who also needed her nappy changing. Not the best way to greet your supervising social worker.

CHAPTER FOUR

FIRST REVIEW – WHAT HAD I AGREED TO?

'And you prefer looking after a baby rather than an older child?' Joy remarked dryly with a smile as she came in.

I liked Joy, we had a good working relationship – much better than the one I had with my previous SSW, Edith.

'Go through to the living room and I'll join you when I've changed her,' I said, and carried Darcy-May upstairs.

She cried throughout the whole process, getting angrier and angrier, as babies can, and I wondered what Joy was making of all this.

Once I'd finished and Darcy-May was clean and dry, I carried her and the bag containing the soiled nappy downstairs.

'I'm just getting her a bottle!' I called to Joy as I passed the open living-room door on my way to the kitchen. I dropped the bag outside the back door for disposing of later and began warming the bottle of milk by running it under the hot tap. My untouched sandwich lay on the plate where I'd left it.

'Is there anything I can do?' Joy asked, coming into the kitchen.

'If you could hold Darcy-May I can make us a drink,' I said.

'Sure.'

I gave Darcy-May to Joy and she cried all the louder. Joy tried to comfort her as I filled the kettle and finished warming the bottle of formula. 'Tea or coffee?' I asked.

'Tea, please, but only if you're making one.'

'Yes, I am.'

'And if that's your lunch you'd better eat it,' Joy said, nodding to the sandwich. 'I'll feed Darcy-May if you like.'

I gave her the bottle of formula and she carried Darcy-May into the living room. I followed with the mugs of tea and my sandwich on a tray. It was a long time since breakfast and I was feeling a bit light-headed from not eating and drinking, so I was grateful for Joy's help. A good SSW like Joy will offer a little practical help where appropriate, rather than just supervising.

We settled in the living room, and once I'd eaten my sandwich and Darcy-May had finished her bottle Joy passed her to me and drank some of her tea. She then took her laptop from her bag and began the more formal part of her visit. The carer's SSW is expected to visit them at least every four to six weeks, more often if necessary, plus two unannounced visits a year. During their visit the carer updates the SSW on the child or children they are fostering, and they ask questions and observe the carer with the child to make sure they are fostering to the required standard. They give advice and direction where necessary as well as discussing the carer's training needs. All foster carers have to attend a set number of training sessions per year, and experienced carers are expected to facilitate some training too.

I told Joy about the routine I was trying to establish with Darcy-May and that the midwife had visited earlier. She made notes on her laptop as I spoke and then checked that the Moses basket, currently in the living room, was suitable and met current safety standards. She asked about pets and I confirmed there was just Sammy and went over the steps I was taking to keep him away from Darcy-May. 'He's never left alone with her,' I emphasized. 'And at present he is scared of her so won't go anywhere near.'

Joy checked the baby monitor and then I stayed in the living room with Darcy-May as she looked around the downstairs. SSWs are expected to look in all rooms in the house at every visit. While she was in the kitchen she checked the sterilizing unit and the area where I prepared food, and opened the fridge door. Darcy-May was sound asleep now so I settled her in the Moses basket and went upstairs with Joy to my bedroom to show her where the basket stood at night. I then left Joy to check the other rooms while I returned downstairs to Darcy-May.

Presently Joy joined me and we continued the meeting. She didn't really have anything new to tell me in respect of Darcy-May but said the care plan was adoption, as there was no one in the extended family to look after her, which is usually considered first. She said she didn't think it would take the permanency team long to find a suitable adoptive family. There is a waiting list of approved adopters wanting a healthy baby. It would just be a matter of matching. Joy finished by arranging a date for her next visit in a month's time, although I would be updating her regularly by email and phone in the interim, as she would me.

* * *

That evening Kirsty, Adrian's fiancée, stopped by to see us all – but mainly to see Darcy-May. She stayed for dinner, which was nice, and we talked about their wedding, among other things. Kirsty is a teacher, and a lovely person; kind, caring and sensitive. She and Adrian have been dating since their student days and I thought they made a great couple – well suited.

That night and the next Darcy-May was restless, which was only to be expected. But the week flew past and by the end of it I felt we were in something of a routine. I took her up for a bath at around 8.30, then fed her and settled her in the Moses basket in my bedroom around 9 p.m. I then spent time with Adrian and Paula and also caught up on household chores and writing. Around 11 p.m. I got changed ready for bed but didn't go to sleep until Darcy-May woke for her next feed, which was usually around midnight. She then slept through until about 3 a.m., when I fed and changed her again. From then she usually slept until 5.30 or 6. A newborn baby only has the stomach capacity to take enough feed for about two to three hours. She went back to sleep and I showered and dressed.

I was taking lots of photographs and short video clips – some for me, but mainly to pass on to the adoptive family. It would form part of Darcy-May's Life Story Book; a record for her new parents, and to share with her once she was old enough.

Lucy and family came for lunch on Sunday and the following week the health visitor, Judy Preston, paid us a call but phoned first. It was mid-morning and Darcy-May was awake and content, having just had her bottle.

I showed Judy into the living room where we discussed Darcy-May's routine – feeding and sleeping – then she weighed her. She was six pounds four ounces, which was good. Not only had she made up her birth weight, but she'd gained three ounces. Judy entered the information on her laptop and in the Red Book. She asked me how I was feeling and if there was anything I needed help with, adding, 'I don't suppose there is, as you're an experienced foster carer.'

'I need sleep,' I said with a smile.

'Yes. Get it when you can is my advice. Most babies can manage five hours at night when they are three months old, which is often seen as sleeping through the night.'

'Sounds good to me,' I said.

She knew Darcy-May was going for adoption and asked me when that would be.

'I don't know yet,' I said. 'But I would guess within a year.'

'You'll miss her when she's gone.'

'We certainly will. She's only been with us a short while, but already we love her,' I said, and ridiculously I felt my eyes fill.

'Ah, bless you,' she said kindly.

We talked a bit about fostering and having to say goodbye to the child, then she updated the Red Book. She said there was no need for her to visit again unless I wanted her to, as I could start attending the baby clinic at my doctor's to have Darcy-May weighed and checked. Before she left, she gave me a leaflet about vaccinations that began when the baby was eight weeks old.

That afternoon Lucy stopped by with Emma. She remarked that I was looking very well.

'Thank you, love. I feel good.'

I was still missing my mother dreadfully, as we all were, but looking after Darcy-May (as well as everything else that was going on) didn't give me time to fret or feel down for long. My mother, like my father, had always been very positive in their outlook and I tried to be like them.

I had begun taking Darcy-May out for a while each day, either shopping or just for a short walk. It was April and the weather was improving. While shopping, I bought my family an Easter egg each, as Lucy wanted to do a little Easter egg hunt for Emma. She was too young to know what it was all about, but we'd all have some fun.

An email arrived from Shari with details of Darcy-May's first review, to be held the following week. All children in care, regardless of their age, have regular reviews. The first takes place within four weeks of the child being placed in care. The social worker, foster carer, the foster carer's support social worker and any other adults closely connected with the child meet to ensure that everything is being done to help the child, and that the care plan (drawn up by the social services) is up to date. Very young children don't usually attend their reviews, but older children are expected to. They are chaired and minuted by an independent reviewing officer (IRO) who is unconnected with the social services. Shari asked that the review be held at my house. Often they are held at the council offices or the child's school.

I made a note of the time and date in my diary, then, while Darcy-May slept, I filled in the online forms for the review I was expected to complete as the foster carer:

details of Darcy-May's routine, sleeping and feeding, and development to date. There were questions about contact with family and friends where I just typed *Not applicable* or *None*. The social worker and IRO saw the form and it would be part of the review. I would also be asked to speak at the review.

The rest of the week disappeared in a round of feeding and changing Darcy-May. I also went to the park with Lucy and Emma.

I felt I had relaxed into looking after Darcy-May and was enjoying it. Adrian had been right. Compared to the challenges that some children bring – a sibling group or an angry aggressive child with very challenging behaviour – this was easy. I wasn't expecting any surprises at the review and assumed my present routine would continue, probably until we began the introductions to the adoptive family – many months away yet.

We had our Easter egg hunt on Sunday and I made us lunch. It was great having all the family together, including Kirsty and Lucy's partner, Darren.

'Nana used to love our Easter egg hunts,' Paula said. She got out some old photograph albums and we all enjoyed a trip down memory lane. I knew how fortunate we were to have so many happy memories. Some families don't have this.

The following Tuesday at 11 a.m. I welcomed Shari, Joy, Judy and Ashley Main, the IRO, into my home for the review. The number attending a review can vary. There are sometimes family present, a teacher, psychologist, nurse and so forth, depending on the child's circumstances. This was a relatively small review. We were holding it in the living room, where Darcy-May slept in the Moses basket. Everyone admired her as they came in.

I made coffees and teas and set them on the small occasional table with a plate of biscuits. Sammy, our cat, was outside in the garden enjoying the sunny spring weather.

'Are we waiting for anyone else?' the IRO asked, opening his laptop.

'No,' Shari said.

'No family coming?' the IRO checked.

'No,' Shari confirmed.

As is usual at the start of these meetings, the IRO asked us to introduce ourselves as he noted down who was present. He then thanked us for coming and said this was the first review for Darcy-May. He gave her date of birth and the date she came into care. The IRO is sent details of the case prior to the review. He asked me to speak first and at that moment Darcy-May woke with a loud cry. I picked her up and she stopped crying so I sat with her in my arms as I spoke. I said she'd been with me three weeks now, having come straight from hospital. That she was feeding well and putting on weight. I had the Red Book and my notes to hand and read out her weight, and the days the midwife and health visitor had seen her.

'So she is progressing as she should be?' the IRO asked as he typed.

'Yes,' I said.

'Does she have any underlying health issues?'

'Not as far as I know,' I said, and glanced at Shari.

'The hospital gave the baby a clean bill of health before they discharged her,' Shari said. 'We're awaiting the results of the heel-prick test.'

Darcy-May began to cry. 'I'll get her a bottle,' I said. 'I won't be a minute.'

I left the room, taking Darcy-May with me, and they waited until I returned before continuing.

'Has Darcy-May had any accidents or illnesses?' the IRO asked me. It was a standard question.

'No,' I replied.

The IRO has a checklist they work through at reviews, designed to give a picture of how the child is doing in care, but many of the usual questions wouldn't apply to a baby; for example, those about friendships, hobbies and school. We sat quietly waiting as he went through the form on his laptop, checking boxes; the others were looking at Darcy-May, as I was.

'Do you have everything you need to foster Darcy-May?' the IRO asked me at length.

'Yes,' I said.

'Are you aware of the care plan?'

'Yes.'

'And you can foster Darcy-May for as long as necessary?' It was another standard question.

'Yes.'

He thanked me and then asked Joy as my supervising social worker if she would like to add anything. She began by explaining her role, mainly for Judy's benefit: that she supervised, supported and monitored my fostering. She said we were in regular contact and she had visited me the week before, and was happy that Darcy-May was receiving a good standard of care. She said I was a highly experienced foster carer but could ask for help if necessary. She added that she thought I was enjoying looking after a baby, and I nodded.

'So you have no concerns or complaints?' the IRO asked her, which was another standard question.

'No,' Joy confirmed.

Darcy-May had just finished her bottle and I began rubbing her back to wind her. As the IRO typed she let out a burp, surprisingly loud for one so small, and everyone laughed.

'I expect that feels much better,' Judy said.

'My wife tells me off for doing that,' the IRO quipped.

The light atmosphere continued as Judy gave her report. She explained that as a health visitor she worked closely with new parents to support them and advised on matters like breastfeeding and so forth, although she recognized that wasn't necessary in this case. She said she had visited me and the baby the week before when she'd weighed Darcy-May and had discussed her routine.

'Have you visited the birth mother?' the IRO asked.

'No,' Judy replied. 'She will have a follow-up appointment at the hospital for her postnatal check-up.'

The IRO nodded and typed as Judy finished by saying that I could call her if I needed any help or advice, but otherwise I would be attending the baby clinic at my doctor's in future.

'Will you be involved there?' the IRO asked.

'Either me or a colleague. It depends who's on duty.'

The IRO thanked her and then asked Shari to speak. She began by going over some background information: that Haylea was fourteen and hadn't known she was pregnant so hadn't received any antenatal care. That the baby was full term and healthy and was now the subject of a care order. She confirmed the care plan was adoption and the permanency team were actively looking for a suitable match.

'Is it the mother's wishes that her baby is adopted?' the IRO asked.

'Yes,' Shari said. 'She recognizes she is not in a position to raise a child.' She continued to say that the social services had had some involvement with the family but not in recent years. 'Although, given what has happened to Haylea, it raises the question that perhaps there should have been,' she added.

'And the baby's father?' the IRO asked.

'Not known,' Shari replied.

'Because?'

'Haylea isn't disclosing it.'

'Where is the mother now?' he asked.

'She's living at Waysbury Children's Home.'

'And she hasn't seen the baby since giving birth?' the IRO asked.

'No, she didn't want to. However, when I spoke to her yesterday she said she would like to see her once.'

It was said so matter-of-factly, and I was concentrating on Darcy-May, that I almost missed it.

'Haylea wants contact?' Joy asked.

'Yes,' Shari said. 'She wants to see the baby once so she can take some photographs. I am going to try to set up an hour's supervised contact at the Family Centre for this Thursday or Friday. She wants to take photos while she is still small.'

'I have some photos she can have,' I offered, recovering from the surprise.

'Thank you. But Haylea wants to see her daughter. There is no reason why she shouldn't.'

'No,' the IRO agreed. 'It will be supervised?'

'Yes. Haylea asked me if the foster carer can stay too, in case the baby cries, as she won't know what to do,' Shari said. Then, turning to me, she said, 'I told her that should be all right. I will be there at the start of contact and there will be a contact supervisor in the room too.'

'Are you happy to do that?' Joy asked me.

'Yes,' I said. It was expected in my role as foster carer.

'So it's just a one-off contact?' the IRO confirmed.

'Yes,' Shari said.

She continued with her report, although there wasn't much more and nothing I didn't already know. The IRO wound up the meeting by thanking us for coming and set the date for the next review in three months' time. I saw them out. It was only then that what I had agreed to hit me.

CHAPTER FIVE

DIFFICULT

I'd met parents of children I'd fostered in the past. Plenty of times. It was usual and part of the foster carer's role to work with parents. Even if the child wasn't going home to live, I saw the parents when I took them to and from contact and at some meetings. If the care plan was that the child could return home then sometimes contact was in my house or theirs, so we saw a lot of each other.

But this was different to anything I had experienced before and it worried me.

Haylea was fourteen – no more than a child herself – and would be seeing her daughter for the first and last time. There was no chance of her parenting the baby, so wouldn't it have been better for her not to see the baby at all? There was no bond between them, so surely not seeing her would be less painful? Unless she felt this could give her closure. Shari hadn't foreseen a problem – just an hour's contact so Haylea could take some photographs while her baby was still tiny, she'd said. She knew Haylea; I didn't.

My thoughts went to other parents of children I'd fostered who'd had to say a final goodbye. It had been heart-breaking. Tayo, whose story I tell in *Hidden*, was one, as was Faye in *Can I Let You Go?*

Those parents had strong bonds with their children, as they'd been living with them prior to coming into care. So when the social services had decided the children couldn't return home they'd had a goodbye contact. Although it had been very upsetting, it had allowed them to move on with their lives. But Haylea didn't have that bond with her baby, so why put herself through that? I thought, returning to where I'd started.

I forced myself to think about other matters and got on with some work on my computer and then housework, between feeding, changing and playing with Darcy-May. She was awake for longer periods now and didn't always go straight back to sleep after a feed as she had done at first, so I held her on my lap, smiling and talking to her, showing her books and toys and making eye-contact. Bonding with her, as doubtless she was with me. I'd brought the bouncing cradle down from the loft and I sat her in that too sometimes so she could see what was going on.

Very soon the afternoon had passed and Adrian and Paula were returning home from work. We ate together as Darcy-May sat in the bouncing cradle gurgling, and we exchanged snippets of our day. Paula talked about her job. She hadn't been in the post long. It was an administrative position in a manufacturing company a short bus ride away. It involved general office work and paid a modest salary but offered the opportunity for promotion. Adrian worked in a firm of accountants where he'd been for some years and took it in his stride now. He talked about the flat he and Kirsty had bought and were now doing up. They were hoping to have it ready for moving into after their wedding. Most of the decorating was taking place at the weekends, as they both worked full time.

'How did the review go?' Paula asked.

'Fine,' I said. 'Darcy-May will be seeing her mother for an hour later this week.'

That was all I said, and the conversation continued on other topics.

I was probably making too much of the forthcoming contact between Haylea and her daughter, I thought. I have a habit of overthinking and putting myself in other people's shoes and worrying unnecessarily. Haylea was young, resilient, and had requested this contact so would take it in her stride, I told myself. She must have felt it was the right decision or she wouldn't have asked Shari for it. I was the one struggling and I needed to stop it. However, years of fostering had taught me that sometimes plans change and weren't as straightforward as they first appeared.

The following morning Shari telephoned to say she'd arranged the one hour's contact for 1 p.m. on Thursday at the Family Centre. She said she was meeting Haylea there early to run through a few things, then, if everything was all right once I arrived, she'd leave us, although the contact supervisor would remain for the whole hour. Most contact at the Family Centre is supervised.

'Is Haylea all right?' I asked.

'Yes. She may not stay for the whole hour, so if she leaves early just come away.'

'OK.' But I wondered if Haylea was already having doubts.

'I'll see you tomorrow then,' Shari said. 'Make sure you bring everything the baby needs.'

'Yes, of course.'

That night Darcy-May took longer than usual to settle and I put it down to colic. No amount of comforting or pacing the room helped. She cried on and off until around midnight, keeping Adrian and Paula awake. Finally, in the early hours she took a feed and then fell asleep. She woke at 2.30 and 5.30, when I fed and changed her. I was exhausted and, instead of getting up at 6 a.m. as I usually did, I crawled back into bed. When I woke it was 9 a.m. and I felt much better. Darcy-May was awake but not crying. I wondered if in future I should change my routine and instead of getting up at six I should return to bed. There was no reason why I should get up early as I did when I had an older child to take to school.

The house was quiet. Adrian and Paula had gone to work and as I checked my phone I found messages from them. *I fed Sammy and left you to sleep xx*, from Paula. *You were out for the count. Have a good day x*, from Adrian. There was also a good morning from Lucy and a text from a friend.

Feeling human again, I got up, fed, washed and dressed Darcy-May, then propped her on a pillow in the middle of my bed while I got ready. She grinned, chuckled and randomly waved her arms as young babies do. I always talked to her when she was awake and she made baby noises in reply as though she was answering me. She fell asleep on my bed and I took her downstairs and settled her in the Moses basket. She woke around 11.30 and I fed and changed her again, then I began packing what I needed to take with me to contact into what had become known as the baby bag. Bottles, nappies, cream, nappy bags, antibacterial wipes, a fabric book and a rattle – although I'd found that shaking my keys was good for amusing or distracting her.

I left the house at 12.30 to drive to the Family Centre, trying to stay positive. I knew the centre well from having taken other children I'd fostered there. It's a single-storey building about a twenty-minute drive away; a place where children in care can see their parents in a safe and comfortable environment. As well as some offices, there is a kitchen, bathroom, toilets and six contact rooms, each made to look like a living room with carpet, curtains, sofa, table and games and toys for children. Usually, once I've seen the child into the room, I leave them with their parents and the contact supervisor, then return to collect them at the end. Now, at Haylea's request, I would be staying, acting *in loco parentis*, responsible for and looking after Darcy-May.

As I drew up and parked outside the Family Centre I felt my pulse quicken. All manner of scenarios flashed through my mind: Haylea weeping uncontrollably, screaming, not wanting to let her baby go, being led away by the manager of the centre who was usually on hand for emergencies if necessary.

I lifted out the portable car seat with Darcy-May still asleep and hung the baby bag over my shoulder. Taking a deep breath, I went up the path to the security-locked main door where I pressed the buzzer. The closed-circuit television camera above me was monitored in the office, and a few moments later the door clicked open and I went in.

'Cathy Glass with Darcy-May to see Haylea,' I said to the receptionist seated at a computer behind a plastic screen to my right.

'She's with her social worker in Purple Room,' she replied. The six contact rooms are identified by the colour they are decorated. 'Sign the Visitors' Book please and you can go in. It's down the corridor, the second room on the left.'

I signed the Visitors' Book and headed towards Purple Room. I knew the layout of the building from having been there many times before. Purple Room was one of the smaller rooms; the larger ones were usually reserved for big families and family reunions. Some children who are in long-term foster care see their family all together a few times a year. I could hear children's laughter coming from some of the rooms. Parents usually try to make contact as happy as possible, although they know that at the end they are going to have to part until the next contact.

The door to Purple Room was closed so I knocked.

'Come in!' Shari called.

I gingerly opened the door and went in. The contact supervisor was sitting at a small table on my left, notebook open in front of her. Straight ahead, Shari was sitting on the sofa beside a teenage girl who I took to be Haylea. Of average height and build, with shoulder-length brown hair, Haylea looked at me warily.

'Hello,' I smiled, and went over.

'Here she is,' Shari said to Haylea as I set the car seat down just in front of her.

Haylea looked at her baby and then at me. I drew up a chair.

'I'm Cathy, Darcy-May's foster carer,' I said, wondering if this hadn't been made clear.

Haylea glanced at the baby again but didn't say anything. Her face was expressionless. She had pale skin and was wearing a viscose floral-print dress that came just below her knees. Rather old-fashioned for someone her age, I thought, compared to what most teenagers were wearing. I didn't know what I was expecting of her, probably someone who looked more sophisticated and older than her years; more streetwise maybe. But Haylea seemed far from mature or streetwise. Indeed, she looked young for her age, like a child wearing an older woman's dress. It was impossible to know what she was thinking and she made no attempt to touch or get close to her baby.

'When was she last fed?' Shari asked me.

'Eleven-thirty, so she'll be waking soon for another feed,' I said, and looked at Haylea.

'It can all be a bit overwhelming to begin with,' Shari said.

But Haylea didn't seem overwhelmed. She wasn't showing any emotion at all. She was looking at me more than the baby.

'I've explained to Haylea that you will stay the whole time and see to what Darcy-May needs,' Shari said.

'Yes, of course.' I threw Haylea a reassuring smile. 'Darcy-May is a lovely name. Did you choose it?'

'Yes,' she said, and maintained eye contact, staring at me.

Shari and I made conversation, talking about Darcy-May's routine and so forth. None of which Haylea joined in with or seemed interested in, although she was concentrating on me. After about fifteen minutes Shari said if we were OK she'd go as she had a meeting later.

'That's fine with me,' I said, and we both looked at Haylea, who gave a small nod.

'How is Haylea getting home?' I asked. For I knew that Waysbury Children's Home, where she was living, was a lengthy bus journey.

'I've booked a cab for her. It brought her here too,' Shari clarified.

I nodded.

Shari stood and, picking up her briefcase, said goodbye and she'd be in touch, then left the room. I sat in the place she had vacated on the sofa, next to Haylea, and looked at the baby. I wasn't sure what to say. Haylea was watching the contact supervisor.

'Did Shari explain about the contact supervisor?' I asked her.

'Yes,' she said in a small voice.

Another silence. 'So, how are you?'

'I get by,' she said quietly.

My heart went out to her. If ever a child looked in need of a mother's love it was Haylea and I now felt silly for worrying about meeting her. She was a young girl who seemed to have lost her way in life. Someone I would have liked to foster and help. Yet what struck me was, given that she was slim, how she had concealed her pregnancy and not known. Surely she would have seen her stomach swelling and realized she'd missed periods?

Darcy-May began to squirm and wriggle in the portable seat as she did when waking. Haylea moved back slightly as if scared of her.

'She's waking up,' I said.

Darcy-May yawned, wriggled some more, then opened her eyes with a cry. Haylea looked very worried. 'It's OK,' I said. I lifted Darcy-May out and sat her on my lap facing Haylea.

I took a bottle of milk from the baby bag, ready. It was still warm. Haylea wasn't looking at Darcy-May but at me, perhaps wondering what I was going to do. I waited a moment and then as Darcy-May pressed her little fist into her mouth – a sure sign she was hungry – I gave her the bottle and she began sucking hungrily. 'Do you want to feed her?' I asked, not knowing if I was doing the right thing in asking.

'No,' she said, and continued to watch me. I wondered again what she was thinking. Certainly nothing could be read in her face. The contact supervisor was looking over and I smiled. Usually they make notes about how the parent is interacting with their child, and then send a report to the social worker after each contact. But there wasn't any interaction between Haylea and her baby.

'I'll take some photographs of you both when she's finished her feed,' I said. 'Do you want to use your phone or shall I take them on mine?'

'I don't have a phone,' Haylea said. 'The social worker is going to get me one.'

'OK. I'll take them on my phone and send them to Shari, who can pass them on,' I suggested.

'I don't want a photo,' Haylea replied.

'No? I thought Shari said you did.' Indeed, that had been given as the main reason for the contact.

'I don't have to have a photo, do I?' Haylea asked in the same quiet voice.

'No, love, of course not.'

Haylea stayed for the whole hour but it didn't get any easier. I tried to engage her in conversation by asking her about school and friends. She said she didn't have a school and shrugged when I asked her about friends. I asked her again if she wanted to hold Darcy-May, but she refused. She didn't touch her during the whole hour, not even her little hand, which most people would have found irresistible. Eventually, when Darcy-May fell asleep, I put her into the portable car seat. There were ten minutes to go.

I tried again to engage Haylea in conversation by asking if she saw her family at all. She replied, 'No.'

'Who do you talk to and share problems with?' I asked, concerned.

Another shrug. 'No one.'

I felt sorry for her and I was also worried. She seemed so alone in the world, but it was hard work, and I was relieved when the hour was up. At exactly two o'clock the contact supervisor put away her notepad and pen, ready to leave, and I repacked the baby bag.

'Do we have to go now?' Haylea asked evenly.

'Yes. I believe you have a cab collecting you.'

We all stood and went towards the door. It's usual for the parent to wait in the room while the carer leaves with the child to avoid any unpleasant or emotional scene outside, but it didn't matter in this case. I doubted Haylea was going to cause a scene when she had to part from Darcy-May. She'd barely looked at her.

'You should wait inside the building until the cab arrives,' I said to her as we went into reception and signed out of the Visitors' Book. I knew that the cab drivers came into the centre to collect the children they transported, for safety's sake. They had the name of the child and all drivers were vetted and police-checked.

'The cab has just arrived,' the receptionist said to us, releasing the door.

A moment later a man came in. 'Car for Haylea Walsh,' he said.

I went with Haylea to the cab where the driver opened the rear door for her to get in. 'Goodbye then, love,' I said. 'Take care of yourself.'

She looked at me but didn't get into the car. 'You are a very nice person,' she said in a small, plaintive voice.

'Thank you, love,' I replied, feeling pretty choked up.

She continued to look at me as if she might be about to say something else but then quietly got into the car.

'Bye, take care,' I said again.

The driver closed her door. She gazed through the side window with the same far-away expression I'd seen in contact, as though she had zoned out of the present and was in another place. I picked up Darcy-May in the car seat and as the cab pulled away I went to my car. Having secured the baby seat in position, I phoned Shari. Clearly, Haylea needed looking after as much as her baby.

CHAPTER SIX

A SHOCK

Shari was on her way to a meeting. 'Is everything all right?' she asked, talking as she walked.

'I've just seen Haylea off in the cab. She didn't want a photo.'

'OK.'

'She seems very withdrawn and alone in the world.'

'Yes, we're helping her. But the contact went all right?' she asked hurriedly.

'I suppose so. She didn't want to hold Darcy-May or have anything to do with her.'

'Perhaps she was overwhelmed. I've got her review tomorrow, so I'll speak to her then. But other than that it was all right? No difficulties?'

'No.' I could tell Shari was in a rush. 'I'll email you later,' I said.

'Thank you.'

I drove home thinking about Haylea. Although there'd been no 'difficulties' as such, I felt great sadness – at what she hadn't said or done. Contained, shut down, emotionally unresponsive were the terms that came to mind. Haylea had seen her baby for the first and last time and had said and done virtually nothing. She'd barely acknowledged Darcy-May, let alone held her or cried. Perhaps Shari was right and Haylea had been 'overwhelmed'. Or possibly she'd seen a likeness to the father in the baby. I assumed her relationship with him was over. A brief teenage romance. It crossed my mind that perhaps Haylea had been raped, but surely she would have told someone? Shari would have talked to her about the father and possibly the police had too, for whether it was rape or consensual, whoever it was had committed a crime by having sex with a minor. Having met Haylea, I could see how easily she could have been taken advantage of. But other than worry about her, there was nothing I could do. It would be for her social worker and the staff at the children's home to protect and support her in the future.

Once home, I unpacked the baby bag, spent time with Darcy-May, then began preparing dinner for later. After Paula and I had eaten, I typed up my log notes and emailed Shari, expressing concern that Haylea had seemed withdrawn, vulnerable, and had no one to talk to. I said I felt she came across as needing a lot of support and maybe counselling. I was sure Shari was doing what she could, but I knew enough of the care system to know that resources were always stretched, so time and money had to be prioritized and would, for example, more likely be allocated to a young child who was being neglected and abused, rather than a teenager who was now in a children's home. I wondered if Haylea would be better off living with a family in a foster placement, but that wasn't for me to say. It was the social worker's decision and foster-care placements are in short supply.

The following day Shari replied, thanking me for my email and saying Haylea did require a lot of support, and had been offered counselling but had refused. They were in the process of identifying a new school for her. I assumed that would probably be the last I heard of Haylea.

April gave way to May and the weather improved. The air warmed, birds built their nests and flowers bloomed. I took Darcy-May out every day, to the park, shopping, sometimes with Lucy and baby Emma. I was having Darcy-May weighed each week at the clinic where I met other mothers with their babies, although they were much younger than me. I did get talking to a similar-aged lady who looked after her grandson during the week so her son and daughter-in-law could work. We exchanged phone numbers and met for a coffee with our babies. I felt I had made a new friend.

Towards the end of May, when Darcy-May was nearly two months old, Joy phoned and asked if I would take another child for a week's respite. The foster carer's mother was ill and lived over a hundred miles away and she wanted to stay with her for a week. I had a spare bedroom; in fact, I had two, as Darcy-May was sleeping in my bedroom, so I agreed.

'Thank you,' Joy said. 'Lea is fourteen and he can be a bit of a handful, but his carer says he responds well to firm boundaries.'

Adrian sighed when I told him and Paula.

'I suppose you need the challenge,' he remarked dryly.

'It's just for a week,' I pointed out.

Paula said very little.

Lea's carer, Gillian, brought him at nine o'clock on Saturday morning. He arrived with a suitcase and bags full of attitude.

'Don't see why I couldn't stay at home,' he grumbled as they came in.

'I've explained it's not allowed at your age,' Gillian said firmly but kindly. I'd met Gillian a few times at training and foster carers' social events.

'I used to stay by myself when I lived with my dad,' Lea moaned.

'It's different in care,' I said, and showed them through to the living room where Darcy-May was in the bouncing cradle.

'A baby. Coochy-coo,' Lea said sarcastically. Flopping down on the sofa, he took out his phone.

'You like babies,' Gillian said.

'Yes, but I couldn't eat a whole one,' Lea quipped.

'The old jokes are the best,' I said to Gillian with a smile.

'He's got plenty of those,' she replied.

I asked her if she wanted a drink, but she said she'd just had breakfast.

'Lea?' I asked. He was concentrating on his phone. 'Do you want a drink?'

'Not fussed.'

'That means no, thank you,' Gillian said. 'Lea will tell you if he wants something. You can't miss it.'

I smiled. I could see that Gillian had established a good working relationship with Lea in the year he'd been with her. As a carer (and parent) you can't take yourself too seriously when it comes to young people. Light-hearted banter can be a good way of deflecting rudeness and see you through a testing situation while getting your message across.

Gillian stayed for about fifteen minutes, then said goodbye to Lea and left to drive to her mother's house. Having seen her out, I returned to the living room and tried to engage Lea in conversation, but he was more interested in his phone.

I knew from the respite information form Gillian had emailed to me that, although Lea's behaviour was still challenging at times, generally he had settled well with her and no longer had violent outbursts, so he was safe to have around babies. Temper and infants don't mix, as accidents can result. The form used for respite care gives basic details of the child or young person: name, age, social worker, school, likes and dislikes, routine, any contact arrangements and so on. It includes a thumbnail history of the young person, from which I'd learnt that Lea's life had been very unsettled and he'd been living with his father until his father had been arrested for drug dealing. He was now in prison. Lea's mother lived with her partner and had community contact with Lea during the school holidays.

Adrian and Paula came downstairs and I introduced them to Lea. He said hi and then continued with whatever he was doing on his phone.

'What are your plans for today, Mum?' Adrian asked.

'I'm not sure. What would you like to do, Lea?'

'Not fussed,' he said, concentrating on his phone.

'Kirsty and I will be continuing decorating the flat,' Adrian said. 'Perhaps Lea might like to come and help? There's plenty to do.' Which was kind of him.

'What sort of thing?' Lea asked, vaguely interested and glancing up from his phone.

'Painting mainly. And I have an IKEA wardrobe I need help assembling. Are you any good at that type of thing?'

'I can paint. I painted my bedroom at my carer's,' Lea said. 'I'll come.'

'Great. I'll just get some breakfast and then we'll be off. Do you want a bacon sarnie?'

'Yes, please,' Lea said enthusiastically, and stood.

Interest aroused, Lea put away his phone and followed Adrian into the kitchen where they made bacon sand-wiches for us all. Adrian, like Paula and Lucy, had been vetted and police-checked for fostering, and Kirsty for teaching, so there wasn't a problem with Lea being in their care for the day. I appreciated Adrian and Kirsty's help. It would make my day that much easier.

On their way back that evening Adrian and Kirsty stopped off to pick up fish and chips, which we ate all together. The following day Lea asked Adrian if he could help them again and he agreed. That evening I made a large spaghetti bolognese for us all, which I knew from the respite information form was one of Lea's favourite meals. Later he moaned when I said it was time for him to go to bed, but overall I felt the weekend had gone well, thanks to Adrian and Kirsty.

The following week I took Lea to and from school each day in my car. It was an hour on the bus from my house and he was saying he didn't want to go to school as it was too far. He used the bus when he was at Gillian's as it was closer, but even then he sometimes didn't arrive, deciding he would rather spend the day in the town or with his friends. Each evening he moaned about doing his homework, which was tedious, but other than that the week passed without any real incident.

When Gillian collected him on Saturday morning he told me pointedly he was pleased to be returning home. But later I learnt from Gillian that he'd said if she had to go away again, he'd stay with us as he liked spending time with Adrian. He also told her he was going to be a painter and decorator when he left school!

The following week I had to take Darcy-May to the clinic for her first vaccination. It was a six-in-one vaccine to protect her against serious illnesses, including diphtheria, hepatitis B, polio, tetanus and whooping cough. I was dreading it. As any parent or carer with a baby knows, it's heart-breaking to have to hold your baby on your lap and try to distract them as they are injected. Of course it hurts and they cry and look at you accusingly as they don't understand it's for their own good. While I soothed Darcy-May, the nurse entered the details of the vaccine in the Red Book. By the time we left, Darcy-May had stopped crying. The next vaccine was in four weeks' time.

On Saturday Tilly Watkins with her best friend Abby came to see us. It was a pleasant surprise. I'd fostered Tilly the year before and I tell her story in *A Terrible Secret*. I was delighted to hear all their news, although they didn't stay for long. They were in the middle of exams but had wanted a break from studying. Tilly had often taken breaks from studying when she'd been living with me – too many. Paula was in and spoke to them and they thought Darcy-May was 'so cute' and 'amazing'. They said they'd visit again once their exams had finished the following month.

Also the following month – in fact, in two weeks' time – it was Adrian and Kirsty's wedding. On Sunday Kirsty's mother summoned me by text for afternoon tea and *to run through the wedding arrangements one last time – make sure we all know what we're doing and I haven't missed anything*. I doubted she had missed anything, but I was happy to go. I took Darcy-May and met Adrian and Kirsty there. Paula was out with a friend. Andrea, Kirsty's mother, was clearly anxious as the big day approached, but she'd done a good job of organizing everything; I told her so and that everything would go to plan. What had started off as quite a small and simple affair had become rather grand, with over a hundred guests. I showed Andrea a photo of the outfit I was wearing and she nodded approvingly. Kirsty and Adrian had already seen it.

On Monday morning I got up feeling very blessed. Life was good. Adrian was getting married to a lovely girl, Lucy was happily settled with her partner, Darren, and I had become a grandmother. Paula was enjoying her job and we were all in good health and had enough money to live on. I knew how lucky we were. I missed my mother but consoled myself that she'd had a long and happy life and was now with my father. I was expecting the week ahead to run smoothly, but then I was ejected from my cosy world by a ring on the doorbell.

It was after lunch and I'd just settled Darcy-May in her cot in my bedroom for a nap and was about to do some work on the computer. Now she was two months old she'd outgrown the Moses basket, so I'd begun using the cot and had returned the Moses basket to the loft. I was in the front room with the baby monitor beside me and had just opened the file I needed on my computer. I wasn't expecting anyone, but sometimes a friend or neighbour dropped by if they saw my car on the drive. Usually I didn't mind, but now I had some work to do so I'd have to keep their visit short.

But it wasn't a friend or neighbour. I opened the front door to find Haylea standing there!

'Good grief! What are you doing here?' I asked, shocked. She wasn't even supposed to know my address.

'I don't know,' she said in a small voice. She looked pale and drawn; a complete contrast to Lea, who was the same age and so full of life.

'Are you alone?' I asked, looking past her to the street.

'Yes. I'm sorry, I shouldn't have come.' She turned and was about to go.

'Haylea, no, wait, love. What's the matter?'

She stopped and looked at me.

'Does your social worker know you're here?'

She shook her head.

'Did you come to see Darcy-May? If so, you will need to speak to Shari to arrange another contact.'

'I came to see you.'

'Why?'

She paused and put her hand to her head. 'I don't feel so good. It was hot on the bus.'

She didn't look well and I could hardly send her back like this.

'You'd better come in,' I said.

Steadying her arm, I took her through to the living room and then fetched her a drink of water. I waited while she drank some. 'I won't be a moment,' I said. 'I need to get the baby monitor.' I brought it in from the front room and placed it unobtrusively on the corner table, then sat in a chair opposite her.

She finished the water and handed me the glass. 'Thank you,' she said. She was wearing a similar-style dress to the one she'd worn at contact, over which was a long, shapeless cardigan with pockets.

'I expect you got a bit hot and dehydrated on the bus. Are you feeling better?'

'A little.'

I looked at her carefully. 'Haylea, how did you know where I live?'

'The hospital told me. I think it was a mistake. I have a mobile phone now and someone from the hospital phoned me to make an appointment. They said, "Are you Haylea Walsh of – ?" and read out your address. I remembered the street and then saw your car with the baby seat in it so I thought it might be you.'

It was feasible. I'd experienced similar accidental breaches in confidentiality before from professionals connected with a case, as have other foster carers.

'You went to a lot of trouble to find me,' I said.

She nodded.

'Why are you here?'

There was just Darcy-May and me in the house and I could see Haylea's eyes travelling around the room. She came from a family with a history of criminal activity. Had she come to rob me or snatch Darcy-May?

She hadn't replied but was now staring at me. 'Now you're feeling better I think you'd better go, love,' I said. 'I'll call your social worker. Do you have enough for the bus fare?'

'No, please don't make me go,' she said, and burst into tears.

CHAPTER SEVEN

HAYLEA

I couldn't just send Haylea out of the door crying. I passed her some tissues and tried to comfort her as best I could. Darcy-May was still asleep upstairs and I could hear little snuffling sounds coming through the monitor. Haylea must have been able to hear them too, but she didn't show it. I felt sorry for her, but at the same time I needed to protect Darcy-May.

'Can I just stay for a bit?' she asked pitifully, drying her eyes.

'Why, love?'

'You seem nice and have a nice home.'

'Thank you, but you're being looked after at Waysbury, aren't you?'

'I suppose so.'

I would have found it more acceptable if Haylea had said she'd come to see Darcy-May, but that didn't appear to be her motive. In fact, I wasn't sure what her reason was for coming.

'I was watching you at the Family Centre,' she said after a moment. 'I could tell you were a kind person and a good mother by the way you were with the baby.'

'You know Darcy-May won't be staying with me?' I checked. 'She will be found an adoptive family.'

'Yes, I know. The social worker told me. I don't want her.'

I was taken aback by the bluntness of her reply. Usually mothers fought to keep their children, and if they did have to give them up for adoption, it was very painful and took them a long time to come to terms with their loss. Haylea didn't appear to have any bond with Darcy-May, but I would have expected her to have felt something – regret? Remorse?

'The adoptive family will love and care for her,' I said.

'I wish you could have adopted me. I would have liked you as my mother.'

'Why do you say that? You barely know me.'

'I didn't really have a mother. Not a proper one. She wasn't there for me. I wish I'd been taken into care and had come to live with someone like you.' She began to cry again.

My heart went out to her, but I was limited in what I could offer. I wasn't fostering Haylea, I had very little information about her past and, strictly, she shouldn't have been here at all. I passed her more tissues, then got her another glass of water.

'I really think you need to talk to your social worker,' I said. 'Shari was going to refer you to a therapist.'

'I don't want to talk to a stranger,' she said, her eyes filling again. 'I think I will just kill myself. It will be easier.'

'No, you won't,' I said, really worried now. 'With help, you will come through this dark time.'

'No one can help me.' She wrung her hands in her lap. 'I don't want to live any more.' More tears slid down her cheeks.

I put my arm around her, but she tensed so I took it away again. Not everyone feels comfortable being hugged.

'Haylea, love, I know you're down right now, but with help you will get better.'

'I won't, I've felt like this for ages. I don't want to live any more.'

Darcy-May had begun to stir. I could hear her through the monitor slowly waking, and I knew it wouldn't be long before she was fully awake and crying.

'What can I do to help you?' I asked Haylea gently.

'Nothing. No one can.'

Haylea was clearly in despair. When I'd seen her at contact she'd been silent and withdrawn, holding it all in; now, for whatever reason, it was coming out.

'Has something happened to make you feel this way?' I asked her.

'Don't know.'

'Perhaps it's postnatal depression. Have you been to the hospital for your check-up?'

'Yes.'

'Did you tell them you were feeling very low?'

'No. I was like this before.'

'And you've never told anyone?'

She shook her head.

'Have you got any friends you can talk to?'

'No. No one likes me. I'm a nasty little slut.'

'Don't say that, love,' I said, shocked.

'But it's true.'

At that moment Darcy-May's murmuring turned into a cry, signalling she wanted to be up. I knew if I left her, her cries would quickly escalate. 'I need to fetch Darcy-May,' I said. 'Then I'll phone your social worker and let her know you're here.'

Leaving Haylea in the living room, I quickly went upstairs, lifted Darcy-May from her cot, then returned to the living room. Darcy-May wasn't due for a feed yet and didn't need her nappy changed, so I put her in the bouncing cradle close by me. Haylea gave her a cursory glance, but that was all.

'Do the staff at Waysbury know you're here?' I asked her, concerned.

'No. They don't care.'

'I'm sure they do care. Where do they think you are?'

She shrugged.

'I'd better let them know, then I'll call your social worker. Do you have the number of Waysbury?'

'Yes. They put it in my phone.' She took her phone from the pocket of her cardigan and gave it to me.

I opened her contacts list. There were just two numbers: that of Waysbury and her social worker. Haylea had only recently been given the phone, but I was surprised she had so few contacts, compared to the number the average young person has.

I added the number of Waysbury Children's Home to my phone and gave Haylea's back to her. She sat quietly, watching me, as I called Waysbury. It went through to answerphone and a recorded message: 'I'm sorry no one is available to take your call. Please leave your name, number and a short message and someone will get back to you as soon as possible.'

'It's Cathy Glass,' I began. 'I'm a foster carer. Haylea Walsh is with me. Can someone phone me, please? She's upset. I'll call her social worker too.'

Haylea was still watching me, not Darcy-May, who was softly chuntering and waving her arms endearingly as babies do. I called Shari's mobile, but that too went through to voicemail, so I left a similar message.

I needed advice as I couldn't just send Haylea off when she was upset and talking about killing herself. If no one returned my call within the next fifteen minutes I would call the duty social worker.

'Can I have a biscuit?' Haylea asked in a small, child-like voice.

'Yes. Have you had lunch?'

'No.'

'Do you want a sandwich?'

'Yes, please.'

'What filling would you like? Ham, cheese, Marmite or peanut butter?'

'Cheese.'

'You can come with me while I make it,' I suggested, not wanting to leave her unattended for any length of time.

Haylea came with me as I carried the bouncing cradle with Darcy-May in it through to the kitchen, where I set her down to watch. Darcy-May liked to be where I was. Haylea stood a little way off also, watching me as I prepared her sandwich.

'You've got a nice kitchen,' she said.

'Thank you.'

It was nothing unusual, but then these things are relative and I'd no idea what the kitchen at her home was like. Perhaps it was dirty and unkempt or perhaps Haylea was just trying to please me; she seemed to want to be liked.

I made us both a mug of tea and we returned to the living room, with Haylea carrying the tray and me Darcy-May. She was still content to sit in the bouncing cradle where she could see what was going on. As Haylea ate her sandwich and I sipped my tea my mobile rang. It was one of the staff at Waysbury.

'We got your message. Why is Haylea with you? Does she know you?'

'Not really. I am fostering her baby. We met at contact once, but it seems the hospital gave her my address. I'm not sure why she came here.'

'When is she coming back?' the member of staff asked.

'I think she needs to come back now,' I replied. 'She shouldn't really be here – it's unauthorized contact – but she seems very low.'

'Why?'

'I don't know exactly, but she's been through a lot.' I was surprised I had to point this out.

'Can she come back on the bus? She knows we're doing her a birthday tea.'

'Birthday tea? Is it her birthday?' I asked, astonished, glancing at Haylea, but she just looked at me, expressionless.

'Yes. Today.'

'She didn't say anything to me,' I said. I could have wept. When you think of the fuss that is made of most children and young people on their birthdays, and how happy they are. Yet here was Haylea talking about ending her life, having not even acknowledged it was her birthday.

'Tell her to come back when she's finished there,' the member of staff said. I felt she hadn't really got the measure of this. Some staff in children's homes are experienced, but others aren't.

'I don't feel comfortable sending Haylea on the bus,' I said. 'Can someone there come and collect her?'

'Not really. We're very short-staffed. There's only two of us here at present. Can you bring her?'

'Yes, I could. Is there someone there she can talk to about her problems?'

'She can talk to any of us.' Which isn't quite the same thing.

'Does she have a key worker?'

'Yes, but it's her day off.'

'I'll bring her back shortly,' I said, and finished the call.

'Haylea, why didn't you tell me it's your birthday, love?' I asked her.

'It doesn't mean anything, and bad things happen on my birthday.'

'Like what?'

'I can't tell you.'

'You mean at home?'

She shrugged.

'They are making you a birthday tea, so that's nice, isn't it?'

'I guess,' she said despondently.

'Have you had any presents and cards?'

'They are going to give me one tonight.'

'OK.'

It was dreadfully sad. Had I been fostering Haylea, my family and I would have bought her presents and cards and done something special to mark the day. As I wasn't fostering her, I hadn't paid any attention to her date of birth on the placement information form. But while my heart went out to Haylea and I felt sorry for her, she wasn't really my responsibility and she needed to go back to Waysbury.

'I'll give Darcy-May a bottle and then take you home,' I said gently.

'Not home, but to Waysbury,' she corrected.

'Yes, that's what I meant.'

I fetched a bottle of formula from the kitchen. As Darcy-May fed I asked Haylea about Waysbury and who she felt she could talk to there. I hadn't been overly impressed with the member of staff I'd spoken to, but she may have been inexperienced or very busy. Haylea said that the staff didn't really have time to talk as they were always dealing with a crisis. It seemed that many of the other residents demanded a lot of attention. 'Some do drugs and fight,' she said. 'Some don't come back at night. The police are always coming. I hide in my room.'

'Oh dear.' I sympathized.

I could imagine Haylea – quiet and self-effacing – hiding in her room when trouble erupted, and generally not getting her fair share of attention. And again, I wondered if she wouldn't be better off in a foster home with a family to look after her.

Once Darcy-May had finished her bottle, I told Haylea I would need to change her before we set off. 'Do you want to use the bathroom? If so, I'll show you where it is.'

She came with me upstairs and as she went to the toilet I went into my bedroom, where I laid Darcy-May on the changing mat in the centre of my bed. Before I changed her, I quickly took a birthday card from my emergency supply and signed it *Best Wishes, Cathy and family*, then put in a £20 note. It was the best I could do at short notice.

I heard the toilet flush and then Haylea's footsteps along the landing. She stopped outside my bedroom door, which was half open. 'You can come in, love,' I said.

The door slowly opened and Haylea took a couple of steps in. She stood quietly to one side, looking around as I finished changing Darcy-May. 'You have a lovely bedroom,' she said.

'Thank you. Is your room at Waysbury nice?'

'It's OK.'

I finished changing Darcy-May and we went downstairs, where I gave Haylea the birthday card. 'There's a little something for you.'

'For me?' She looked shocked. 'Why?'

'It's your birthday.'

She appeared genuinely overcome.

'Shall I open it?'

'If you want to, or save it to open at your birthday tea. It's up to you.'

'I'll save it,' she said, and a tiny smile crossed her face.

'OK, love. Now we'd better be off.'

As I put on my shoes and threw the baby bag over my shoulder, my gaze fell on the computer in the front room. So much for an afternoon of working! I thought. And I still didn't know why Haylea had come.

CHAPTER EIGHT

IN TROUBLE

'Will I be in trouble for not telling someone I was going out?' Haylea asked me as I drove to Waysbury.

'I don't know. What are you supposed to do?'

'Tell someone. It's one of the rules.'

'It's to keep you safe,' I said.

'There are other rules, but I don't break them.'

'Good.'

'You're not allowed to smoke, drink alcohol or take drugs,' she said. 'And we have to respect each other and their property, and not go into their rooms without asking first.'

'That's similar to the rules foster carers have. They are to keep everyone in the house safe.'

'That's what the staff said. Usually I'm a good girl and follow them.'

Something about the term 'good girl' on the lips of a fifteen-year-old grated on me, but I didn't comment. I glanced in the rear-view mirror at Darcy-May asleep in her car seat. Haylea was so much more talkative now than she had been at contact. I felt she was opening up.

'Why did you leave Waysbury without telling anyone?' I asked.

She shrugged. 'I woke up feeling pissed off – excuse my language – then I thought of you and what a nice lady you are. So I decided to come and see you. I've been thinking about coming since the hospital gave me your address. I knew if I told someone at Waysbury they would say I shouldn't go.'

I nodded. 'Did you get any birthday cards from your family?'

'No. I don't think they know where I am. I hope I don't get into trouble for not telling anyone I was going out,' she said, clearly worried. 'You get sanctioned if you break the rules.'

'What sort of sanction?'

'You lose privileges and sometimes have to have time out.'

I thought it would be a bit mean to sanction Haylea on her birthday, especially as it appeared that her behaviour was usually good in the home. However, it was obviously worrying her. 'Would you like me to come in and speak to a member of staff and explain?' I offered.

'Yes, please. You are nice to me. No one has ever been this kind to me before.'

I glanced at her, wondering if she was sincere. Had her past life experiences been so dreadful that my small act of kindness put me on a pedestal? I didn't think she had the guile to try to play with my feelings, so I took her comment at face value.

'Don't worry. I'll come in,' I said.

'Thank you.'

Five minutes later I pulled up and parked in the road outside Waysbury. Although I had been to the house before, it was some years ago. Normally I didn't have a reason to come here. It was situated on the far side of town – a large, detached house built in the 1970s, which had been added to and updated over the years. It could take up to ten young people, aged twelve to eighteen, plus residential staff. Everyone had their own bedroom, which now included Wi-Fi.

I got out and went round to the pavement where I lifted out Darcy-May in the car seat. She didn't wake. Haylea joined me on the pavement and looked warily at the house.

'Come on, love, you'll be fine once you're inside. They're doing a birthday tea for you.'

'That's later when everyone is back from school.'

I went first down the front path; the gardens either side – lawn and flowerbeds – were neatly tended. The front door was security-locked and covered by CCTV, so I pressed the bell. No one answered, so I pressed again. Eventually the door was opened by a young woman who looked at me questioningly. 'Yes?'

She was fashionably dressed, with nose piercings, tattoos and braided hair – I wasn't sure if she was a member of staff or a resident until I spotted her ID badge partially covered by her long hair.

'I'm Cathy Glass, foster carer. I phoned earlier. I've brought Haylea back.'

'Thanks,' she said. Then to Haylea, who was standing behind me, 'Come in.'

Haylea didn't move.

'Can I come in?' I asked. 'I'd like to speak to someone responsible for Haylea.'

'There's just me and the manager, Fran, in.'

'I'd like to speak to Fran then, please.'

'Have you got your ID?'

I set down the baby car seat, which was heavy on my arm, and rummaged in my bag for my ID. I'd have thought it was unnecessary as I had Haylea and the baby with me, but I guessed the staff had been told to check all visitors' IDs.

I showed her my card and she opened the door wider.

'Fran's in the office,' she said. 'Can you sign in first?'

I signed the Visitors' Book and then we followed her down the hall to a room on the right. The door was open and another woman sat behind a desk talking on the phone. When she saw us she gesticulated for us to wait as she wouldn't be long. Haylea and I remained by the door. Music could be heard playing loudly from an upstairs room and the member of staff who'd seen us in went up. Apart from the music and some noises coming from the kitchen further along the hall, the rest of the house was quiet. Presumably because most of the residents were at school at this time.

Fran finished on the phone and stood. 'Hi,' she said with a smile. 'I'm Fran Pacton.' She came over, far more confident in her role than the person who had just admitted us.

'I'm Cathy Glass, foster carer.'

'Pleased to meet you. Hello, Haylea. Let's sit down.' Fran closed the door and we sat in the chairs in front of the desk.

'And this must be Darcy-May,' she said.

'Yes,' I replied.

'She's gorgeous.' Fran smiled at her. 'Very cute.' Darcy-May was still asleep and Haylea, sitting beside me, was looking the other way.

'Haylea wanted me to come in as she was worried, having left without telling anyone,' I said. 'She knows she's done wrong.'

Fran turned her attention to Haylea. 'I'm glad you're back now, safe and well. But in future you mustn't leave without telling a member of staff where you're going. We were worried and would have called the police and reported you missing had Cathy not phoned to say you were with her.' Her manner was gentle but firm.

'I'm sorry,' Haylea said remorsefully, meeting her gaze.

'All right. I appreciate you don't normally disappear, but if you want to see your baby again you need to tell us so we can arrange it through your social worker.'

Haylea nodded. Although seeing her baby didn't appear to be her motive for visiting me. She hadn't so much as looked at her; even now, it was Fran who was drawn to Darcy-May, not Haylea.

'I don't want to see her again,' Haylea said after a moment. 'Can I go to my room now?'

'Yes, if you wish. We can talk later,' Fran replied.

Haylea immediately stood. 'Thanks for bringing me back,' she said to me, and left, closing the door behind her.

'Will she be all right by herself?' I asked.

'Aggie – who let you in – is upstairs, she will keep an eye on her.'

'Have you got time to talk?' I asked. 'I am worried about Haylea.'

'So are we. How did she end up at your house?'

'She caught the bus. Apparently the hospital told her my address. She just arrived. She seems so unhappy and alone in the world, with no friends or family. She was talking about not wanting to live any more.'

Fran nodded sombrely. 'She doesn't want contact with any of her family and hasn't really made any friends here yet. She won't engage with her key worker. I've asked her social worker for a referral to the mental-health team.'

'What's happening about school?' I asked.

'She doesn't want to return to her old school, not that she was there very much anyway. We're trying to find her another one, but these things take time. In the meantime I've applied for additional funding for a tutor to come here. One of our lads has some tutoring.'

'Good, but I get the feeling she should be mixing more with her peer group.'

'I agree. Haylea needs the social interaction that comes from school. She spends too much time alone and often in her room. We take her out when we can and she likes to help Cook in the kitchen. She'll be helping her ice her birthday cake later.'

'That's nice.' I smiled weakly.

'Haylea struggles to relate to others her own age,' Fran said. 'And is generally very wary of strangers, but she seems to have taken to you. She told Cook she thought you were a nice lady. In fact, when she returned from contact all her comments were about you, not the baby. Cook found it most odd.'

'She didn't seem interested in Darcy-May at contact or today,' I said. 'She comes across as being a lot older than her years in some respects, but childlike in others.'

'As one of our other girls here put it, it's as though she's been living in a time warp. Haylea acts and dresses more like a middle-aged woman. One of the workers here took her shopping and she wanted long dresses that covered her knees – for "modesty". And she said make-up was for sluts. She didn't have a mobile phone when she arrived, which is unheard of. We sorted one out for her.'

I nodded.

'Haylea is very obedient,' Fran continued. 'She wants to please, so I was surprised when she disappeared this morning. It's completely out of character. I guess the pull of seeing her baby again took over. When I speak to her I'll make it clear if she wants to see Darcy-May again it has to be through her social worker.'

'I don't think that was her reason for coming to see me,' I said. 'She didn't want anything to do with her baby. She won't even look at her. It's as though they're not in the same room. She gravitates towards me, and said she wished I could have fostered her.'

'She told Cook she wished she'd been her mother. Even asked her if she could live with her. It's very sad, but so many of our young people here have attachment issues from not being given a stable, loving home. I'm certain Haylea didn't have much in the way of positive parenting, although there wasn't a lot of social services involvement.'

'I think she's very vulnerable and could easily be taken advantage of.'

'Agreed. Did she talk to you about the father of her baby?' Fran asked.

'No. Has she told anyone here who he is?'

Fran shook her head. 'The only person she talks to is Cook and when she asked her about her boyfriend

Haylea said she'd never had one. I think she is in denial that she has even had a baby.'

I looked at her thoughtfully. 'Yes, you're right. I hadn't thought about it like that, but it would explain why Haylea can so easily ignore Darcy-May and behaves as though she's nothing to do with her.'

'And why she didn't ever go for antenatal treatment,' Fran added. 'The sooner Haylea gets into therapy and starts talking about what happened to her, the better.'

I agreed.

The phone on Fran's desk began to ring. 'Excuse me, I need to take this,' she said.

I waited for a few moments as she talked, but it soon became obvious she would be needed for some time and I'd said what I wanted to. I stood and mouthed that I would go.

'Can you leave me your phone number in case I have to contact you?' she said, covering the mouthpiece, and pushed a notepad and pen across her desk.

I wrote down my mobile number and she nodded a thank-you. Picking up the car seat, I left. Darcy-May was awake now and would be wanting a feed soon. Once in the car, I sat in the rear where there was more room and gave her a bottle, then I strapped her into her car seat. She grinned and gurgled. I smiled and kissed her nose. As I was getting out to sit in the driver's seat my phone rang. Shari's number came up, so I answered the call as I got in.

'Is Haylea still with you?' Shari asked.

'No, I've just returned her to Waysbury.'

'I got your message. What happened?'

I explained how she had arrived at my house and what she'd said, emphasizing that she had seemed very low and had talked about ending her life. 'And it's her birth-day!'

'Yes, I know, I've sent her a card. Haylea has been offered counselling but is refusing. Perhaps she's changed her mind. I'll give Fran a call now.' As Haylea's social worker, Shari would be in regular contact with Waysbury, just as she was with the foster carers of the children she was responsible for. 'And on another matter, I've just heard from the permanency team,' she said. 'They've identified two prospective adopters who look like good matches for Darcy-May. So that's something.'

'Good. Will you tell Haylea?'

'Not at this stage. She will be offered a goodbye contact, but that's further down the line. I'll speak to Fran now and see how Haylea is.'

We said goodbye. I had mixed feelings that two 'good matches' had been found for Darcy-May. While it was important she was settled with her permanent family as soon as possible, my family and I would obviously miss her when she went. She was already part of our family. However, that's the nature of fostering. While some babies and children stay with their first foster carer long term, most do not. They either return home, go to live with a relative or are adopted. It's for this reason that some people who would like to foster don't. Adoption is different in that it's permanent, and once the adoption order has been granted, the parents and child have the same legal rights and responsibilities as if the child had been born to them.

Driving home, it wasn't Darcy-May I was worrying about – it would be many months before she had to leave – it was Haylea. Darcy-May would be given a new life and would be too young to remember a time before that, but Haylea was very different. Her past was still with her and she was in a very bad place right now and needed help. I hoped that Shari and Fran could persuade Haylea to go for counselling. I also hoped that she had a nice birthday tea. She deserved it, poor girl.

My thoughts stayed with Haylea for the rest of the day, although I didn't expect to hear from her again, at least not so quickly.

The following morning my mobile rang and Waysbury's number came up. I immediately feared the worst and thought Haylea must have run away again and they were calling to see if she was with me.

'Cathy speaking,' I said.

'Hi. I'm Dylis, Haylea's key worker at Waysbury.'

'Yes? How can I help?'

'Haylea is with me now and would like to talk to you. Is that OK? She just wants to thank you.'

'Yes, sure,' I said, relieved.

Haylea came on the phone. 'Hi, Cathy,' she said in her small, childlike voice. 'I want to say thank you for my birthday card and present. It's so kind of you.'

'You're welcome, love. Did you have a nice evening?'

'Yes, I did. It was wonderful. I was so touched. Everyone was nice to me. I had a party with jelly and ice-cream and a huge birthday cake, which I helped ice. Everyone sang "Happy Birthday", even the staff, and they cheered as I blew out the candles. Then we played some games. I've never had a birthday party or presents like that before. I am lucky.'

A lump rose in my throat. Bless her, I thought. I would like to say it was the first time I'd come across a child who'd never celebrated their birthday or been given presents, but unfortunately that's not so, and it's heart-breaking.

'I'm glad you had a good evening,' I said.

'I did. I've got my cards on a shelf in my room. You have all been so kind to me. I don't deserve it.'

'Of course you deserve it,' I said, but the line had gone quiet. Then Dylis came on.

'Haylea is a bit emotional,' she said. 'I'll have to go.'

'OK. Give her my love.'

'I will.'

For the rest of the day Haylea's words rang in my ears. Her gratefulness and self-depreciation over something most children took for granted moved me deeply. Again, I wondered what past life experiences had formed her. I hoped her birthday party and other small acts of kindness would show her there were good people out there and life was worth living.

Sadly that wasn't to be. The next day I received a phone call to say Haylea was in hospital, having tried to take her own life.

CHAPTER NINE

HOSPITAL VISIT

It was Fran, the manager of Waysbury Children's Home, who phoned me.

'Haylea took a lot of tablets in a suicide attempt and is recovering in hospital,' she said.

'Oh no. When?'

'Yesterday. She was found in her room by a member of staff. She's awake and talking now and is asking for you.'

'Why me?'

'She wants you to visit her. She's in the children's ward and most of the others there have a parent with them a lot of the time. She wants you to visit like a foster mother. Her key worker and I have been, but we can't stay too long. We just haven't enough staff here. Are you able to see her?'

'Yes, but I won't be able to stay for too long either. I have Darcy-May and I can't take her with me.'

'I think if you just went for a short while it would help her.'

'All right. What happened? When she phoned me yesterday morning she seemed OK and said she'd had a nice birthday.'

'I don't know what triggered it, but after lunch she went to her room and an hour later her key worker found her. We're looking into where she got the tablets from and there'll be an enquiry here, although correct procedure was followed. I'll let the ward know you're going.'

'Are any of her family likely to arrive?' I asked.

'No. Haylea has said she doesn't want them told. Shari will have to notify her father as next of kin, but she's going to wait until Haylea is out of hospital in a couple of days.'

'Which hospital is it?'

'The city hospital. Where she had the baby. The children's ward is on the third floor.'

'Yes, I know it. I'll go shortly.'

'Thank you. I'll phone the ward and let them know.'

Poor Haylea, I thought as the call ended. How desperate she must have been to try to end her life. But if I'm honest, I wasn't completely surprised. She was only fifteen and carrying a huge burden that she couldn't talk about. Thankfully she hadn't succeeded in her suicide attempt, and I hoped she would now receive the care she needed to share her pain and set her on the path to recovery. Talking can be very cathartic and many therapies are based on it.

It wasn't appropriate to take Darcy-May with me to the hospital. She would be exposed to germs and also it wasn't fair on Haylea, who could be further upset by having her present and might start to bond with her. I had to find someone to babysit at very short notice. I phoned my daughter Lucy. She was one of my nominated carers, so I could leave a child I was fostering with her for short periods.

'Hi, love,' I said as she answered. 'This is a big ask but can you look after Darcy-May for a couple of hours? Her mother is in hospital and is asking to see me.'

'Yes, bring her here. Is Haylea ill then?'

'She's recovering. She'll be out in a few days. Are you sure it's OK? I'm not stopping you from doing something?'

'No, Darren is here. He's got a day off. It's fine, Mum.'

'Thank you so much. I'll be with you in about half an hour if that's all right.'

'Yes, see you soon.'

I quickly packed the baby bag with bottles of formula and more nappies. The baby seat was still in the car. Before I left the house I emailed Shari and Joy: *My daughter Lucy is looking after Darcy-May for a couple of hours this afternoon so I can visit Haylea in hospital. This is Lucy's address and phone number.* Her details should have been on their system but notifying Haylea's social worker and my support social worker was a precautionary measure. Fostering had taught me it's wise for carers to cover themselves, just in case.

I settled Darcy-May in her car seat and drove to Lucy and Darren's flat. I didn't stay long. I just took her in, said hi, made a fuss of my granddaughter Emma, then ten minutes later I was driving to the hospital. It was strange not having Darcy-May in the back. I kept glancing in the rear-view mirror to check on her before realizing she wasn't there. But my thoughts were mostly with Haylea.

When she'd telephoned yesterday could I have said something that might have made her feel better or at least able to tell someone she was very low? Yet more worryingly, had I inadvertently said something that had sent her on a downward spiral and led to her trying to take her own life? I shuddered at the possibility and thought back to our conversation. I couldn't think of anything I'd said that might have caused her pain. I remembered being moved by her gratitude and humbleness, but I couldn't think of anything that had raised alarm bells with me or I would have told a member of staff at Waysbury straight away.

I parked in the hospital car park, got out and crossed to the main entrance. I went first to the hospital shop where I bought a selection of magazines I thought Haylea might like. If she wanted anything else, I could return. At the end of the corridor I took the stairs to the children's ward and pressed the buzzer. The walls either side of me were brightly decorated with paintings of animals and cartoon characters, just as they were inside the ward too. I'd been here before with children I'd fostered.

It was some moments before anyone answered – they were probably very busy. 'Yes?' asked a female voice.

'Cathy Glass. I've come to see Haylea Walsh,' I said into the grid.

'Are you a relative?'

'No. I'm a foster carer. The manager of the care home where Haylea is staying phoned me. I understand Haylea is asking to see me. She's fifteen,' I added.

'Just a minute.'

It went quiet and then the door was released. I stepped in and used the hand sanitizer on the wall to my right. A large painting of a giraffe looked down at me, its head nearly touching the ceiling. I went to the nurses' station.

'I'm Cathy Glass. I've come to visit Haylea Walsh. Which room is she in?'

'Bay C, down there on the left,' the nurse said, pointing.

'Thank you.'

I went along the corridor, past more painted pictures of animals, and into Bay C. There were four beds, two on each side. I saw Haylea straight away in a bed to the right and closest to the window. She saw me too. She pulled herself further up the pillows and, smiling, took out her earphones.

'Hello, love,' I said, pulling up a chair.

'Oh Cathy, you came! Thank you so much. I didn't know whether you would come after all the trouble I've caused.' My instinct was to kiss and hug her, but she gave no indication she wanted that, although she was clearly glad to see me.

'I'm pleased you're looking so well,' I said. She did look well, relaxed, and there was no sign of the trauma she'd suffered the day before. 'I bought you these magazines,' I said, putting them on the bed. 'I wasn't sure what you liked. I can go down to the shop if you need anything.' There was fruit in a bowl, a box of tissues and a book on the table at the end of the bed.

'Fran brought me some things,' she said.

'Have you got everything you need? Toothbrush, face flannel and so on?'

'Yes. They're in this bedside cabinet,' she said, pointing. 'And Dylis put some music on my phone.'

'Good.'

'Everyone has been so kind to me. I feel bad for causing them so much trouble. It's nice here. I like it.'

'Do you?' Most young people want to get out of hospital as soon as possible.

'I feel safe here,' she said. 'The doors are locked.'

'Don't you feel safe at Waysbury?' I asked, concerned. 'The outside doors are locked there too.'

'I know, but it's nice here. I can stay in bed if I want. I like being looked after. That girl over there said hello to me, but she had an operation this morning.'

I glanced over. The girl appeared to be a similar age to Haylea. Her parents were either side of her bed and she was awake but pale and drowsy. One of the other beds on the ward was empty, although a child's belongings was on it, suggesting they would be returning soon. In the fourth was a lad with a broken leg. His mother was with him.

'I love all the pictures on the walls,' Haylea said. 'And the food's nice.'

I noticed Haylea hadn't asked where Darcy-May was, but I thought she should know in case she wondered about it later. 'My daughter, Lucy, is looking after Darcy-May while I'm here,' I said. 'I'll collect her on the way back.'

Haylea ignored my comment and changed the subject. 'They let me stay in bed to have my meals,' she said. 'We had fish pie for lunch. Normally I don't like fish, but it was nice. We had apple crumble and custard for pudding. The custard was a bit lumpy, not as good as Cook's, but still nice.'

I smiled. 'I expect you'll be able to return to Waysbury and Cook's food before long.'

'I don't mind staying here,' Haylea said.

I could see that. She was the happiest and most relaxed I'd seen her, and to some extent I understood why. Being a patient had allowed her to return to a childlike state: in bed, given lots of attention, having all her needs met and with no demands being made of her. But it wasn't healthy, and once she was discharged, everything that had driven her to breaking point before would still be out there, waiting.

'Has a doctor from the mental-health team been to see you?' I asked.

'Is that the psychiatrist?'

'Yes. It could be.'

'She came this morning, but I didn't want to talk to her.'

'Why not? She can help you.'

'I don't want her help. The meals come on a trolley,' Haylea said, changing the subject again. 'They bring them to me in bed.'

'OK. But I am very worried about you, as are other people. Why did you take all those tablets?' I asked.

'I didn't want to live.'

'Why not?'

'Sometimes I feel like that. It just comes over me and I go into a very dark place. I'd had a nice birthday, the best ever. Usually bad things happen on my birthday, but this year they didn't. Then it was all over and I knew I'd have to wait a whole year for another birthday. I got very sad.'

'But there are other things in life that can give us pleasure,' I said, saddened she could think this way. 'What bad things happened on your other birthdays?'

'I don't know. Nothing. I shouldn't have told you that.' Her previous happy expression vanished and her face clouded over.

'Haylea, has someone hurt you in the past?' I asked, touching her arm.

She didn't answer.

'You had a baby, love. How did that happen?'

More silence. She began chewing her bottom lip. I didn't want to upset her, but she needed to share this with someone.

'Haylea, if you can't tell me then please talk to the psychiatrist or someone at Waysbury. If someone hurt you then you need to tell.'

'All right,' she said, more to deflect me than from any real agreement. She began talking about the hospital again and how nice the nurses were.

I stayed for an hour, during which time we talked mainly about the hospital routine, then I said I had to go. Haylea looked sad.

'Can't you stay a bit longer?' she asked.

'Five minutes and then I must leave to collect Darcy-May from Lucy.'

It was actually more like fifteen minutes. As I prepared to go, Dylis, Haylea's key worker from Waysbury, arrived, which made my departure easier.

'Take care, love,' I said to Haylea.

'Thanks for coming,' she said brightly. 'I've had lots of visitors!'

I said goodbye to them both and left, no nearer to finding out what had driven Haylea to make an attempt on her life. I understood she'd felt down after having a lovely birthday, but highs and lows are a part of life. We learn to ride them from childhood. I'd seen her switch moods easily and also zone out, but I felt the key to what was really troubling her lay in what she'd said about bad things happening. What were they? Possibly her mother leaving, or something to do with her father, or the father of her baby? I'd no idea.

Still thinking of Haylea, I drove to Lucy and Darren's, where I accepted a cup of tea and stayed for a while, talking to them and playing with Emma while Darren took care of Darcy-May. She was sociable and didn't mind going to others. Lucy asked how Haylea was and I said she was recovering.

'Will you see her again?' Lucy asked. 'If so, I can look after Darcy-May.'

'Thanks, love, but I don't think I will. It hasn't been mentioned and she should be discharged soon.'

'Are you still taking Darcy-May to the wedding?' Lucy asked. Adrian and Kirsty's wedding was in ten days' time.

'Yes. Why?'

'So it will be OK to take Emma?'

'Yes, of course. Kirsty's mother knows we're bringing them.'

'But she's not keen, is she? She's worried about them making a noise.'

'Kirsty and Adrian have invited the children of all their guests, so don't worry. Just take some things to amuse Emma. She'll be fine.'

I was used to taking children to functions, but I could understand Lucy's apprehension. 'Pack a bag of toys for her,' I said. 'But obviously nothing that makes a noise.'

'So not the quacking duck, singing teddy or talking book?' Darren said with a mischievous smile.

'No. Nor this squeaking chick,' I said, giving it a

squeeze. Emma chuckled. I kissed and cuddled her. She was gorgeous.

That evening, when Darcy-May was asleep in her cot, I emailed Shari and Joy with a brief résumé of my visit to Haylea in hospital and also added it to my log. I included that she'd said she felt low after having such a nice birthday and previously bad things had happened on her birthday, although she didn't want to say what. When I read it through before sending I changed it so instead of writing 'she didn't want to say', I put, 'Haylea couldn't talk about what happened,' which seemed to sum it up better. I'd felt she wanted to but couldn't.

On Saturday Adrian had his stag do and went paintballing with friends, followed by a boozy meal. The package included pick-up and drop-off, which was just as well. I normally never hear Adrian come in late at night, but he managed to wake Paula and me as he laughed and talked on his phone, then tripped up the stairs, cursed, apologized and then spent ages flushing the loo. I didn't say anything. It's not every day your son gets married.

The following morning I left him to sleep in and he finally appeared at 3 p.m. 'Did you have a good time?' I asked.

'Ask me tomorrow,' he said. 'I've got a headache.'

I knew that Kirsty and her friends had arranged to go to a nightclub, so I texted her saying I hoped she'd had a nice time. It was late afternoon before she replied. *Yes, thank you*, with an emoji of a woozy face.

The next week, in the run-up to the wedding, was of course dominated by the big day. Kirsty's mother had set up a WhatsApp group some months ago for all the guests. It had become known as the wedding WhatsApp group and was busier than ever. She began a countdown, ticking off the hours to go, interspersed with reminders about arrangements, including if it was raining and where to park if the car park was full. Others in the group replied and with over a hundred guests my phone was constantly buzzing. Eventually I set the group on silent and checked the messages every so often. John, my ex-husband, was coming to the wedding, although he didn't participate in the group. He and his partner had been invited but only he was coming. I didn't know why and I didn't ask. Was I concerned about meeting him again? No. He had left when my children had been very young so it was history now, and nothing would stop me from enjoying my son's wedding.

CHAPTER TEN

I LOVE YOU SO MUCH

Adrian's best man collected him on the morning of the wedding, as they needed to be at the church before us. They both looked super smart in dark-grey three-piece suits bought especially for the wedding. Paula and I went in my car with Darcy-May, and met Lucy and her family at the church. The weather was perfect. The sun shone in a clear blue sky. The air was still, so ideal for outdoor photographs. I fed Darcy-May in the car before we got out and then carried her into the church. I had a spare bottle of milk in my handbag. The arch over the doorway leading into the church was adorned with flowers, as were the aisle and windowsills.

An usher showed us to our seats – front row on the right of the church – while Kirsty's family was being directed to the left, as is tradition. Adrian and his best man were already standing in position at the front. Lucy, Darren and Emma joined us. Emma was wearing a similar dress to Darcy-May: long, lacy, pink – impractical but adorable. It wasn't coincidence; we'd chosen them together. John arrived and, as the groom's father, was shown to the end of our row. He smiled at us, then said a few words to Adrian and the best man before taking his seat. He talked to Darren as we waited, then, when the music changed, signalling the bride had arrived, we all fell silent, stood and watched Kirsty walk down the aisle on the arm of her father.

She looked stunning, magical, in her white full-length, slim-fitting dress trimmed with lace. She was carrying a bridal bouquet of peach flowers the same shade as the bridesmaids' dresses. Her hair was arranged beautifully around a glittering tiara. There were four bridesmaids – two adults (Kirsty's cousins) and their children – plus a little pageboy, who looked so cute in his light-grey trousers, waistcoat and bow-tie. He wasn't at all shy and grinned at everyone as he passed. Kirsty joined Adrian at the front and they smiled lovingly at each other as her father went to sit next to his wife. Kirsty and Adrian's big day had finally arrived.

The vicar began the service: 'Dear friends and family of Kirsty and Adrian, welcome and thank you for being here on this important day. We are gathered together to celebrate the very special love between Kirsty and Adrian by joining them in marriage ...'

I felt so proud and emotional as the service continued, and when they took their vows they gave fresh meaning and added sincerity to the well-known words '... to have and to hold from this day forward, for better, for worse, for richer, for poorer, in sickness and in health, to love and to cherish, till death do us part, according to God'. I stole a glance at John, but he was looking straight ahead.

'... forasmuch as Kirsty and Adrian have consented together in holy matrimony, and have pledged their love and loyalty to each other, and have declared the same by the joining and the giving of rings, by the power vested in me, and as witnessed by friends and family, I now pronounce you husband and wife'.

They kissed and we all clapped. Then they went into the vestry with their witnesses and the photographer to sign the marriage register. They left the church to the song '(Your Love Keeps Lifting Me) Higher and Higher'. Then the congregation followed them out for photographs.

The children had behaved impeccably; the only noise had come from an elderly gentleman occasionally clearing his throat. I felt sure Kirsty's mother would have the video recording she was hoping for. Outside the photographer arranged us in groups to have our pictures taken, some without Darcy-May – at Andrea's suggestion. John was naturally in the family group photos and was placed next to me.

'It all went well,' I said politely.

'Yes,' he agreed.

I'd been very angry with John when he'd first left, but that was years ago, and any animosity I'd felt at the time had long gone, although I hadn't forgiven him for leaving the children and I doubted I ever would.

Once the photographer had finished, it was time to go to the reception, which was being held at a country hotel. I could have gone in one of the limousines, but I'd already explained to Andrea that it would be easier for me to take my car, which had the car seat for Darcy-May. Kirsty and Adrian left first in the white vintage Rolls-Royce decorated with white ribbon and flowers, and we waved them off. The bridesmaids and Kirsty's parents went in a limousine and the rest of us used our cars.

I took the baby car seat into the reception so I didn't have to hold Darcy-May the whole time. There were drinks on arrival and more photographs as the guests mingled. I'd met many of Kirsty's family before at their engagement party and conversation flowed, and then continued as we were shown through to the dining room. It was beautifully adorned with flowers, balloons and decorations that kept the white and peach colour theme going. There was a small top table where Kirsty and Adrian sat and the rest of us were seated at round tables, also beautifully decorated. Paula, Lucy and family were on my table as were some friends of Kirsty's, one who'd come by herself and soon got talking to Paula. The food arrived – three delicious courses with a choice of drinks.

As we'd finished eating, the speeches began with Kirsty's father, Malcolm. It was witty as well as moving and he said some nice things about having Adrian as a son-in-law. Adrian was next to speak and I felt nervous for him, but I needn't have worried. He was well prepared and confident. He said how lucky he was to have found Kirsty and thanked her parents for the wedding, especially her mother, Andrea, who had gone to so much trouble to organize it and had done a fantastic job. He said his only sadness was that his dear nana wasn't here to share in this perfect day, for she would have enjoyed it so much. He proposed a toast to her and Grandpa – 'the best grandparents ever', he said. I felt my eyes fill.

The best man also made a speech, which included reminiscing about their student days, much to Adrian's embarrassment. We were then shown through to another room where we would spend the evening. A children's entertainer was already in place to keep the little ones amused and then later there was a disco. John didn't stay for that and left soon after the meal. He came to say goodbye and said he'd see Adrian and Paula again soon. Paula and I stayed until the end, as did Lucy and family, dancing, talking, laughing and generally having a fantastic time. Darcy-May slept through a lot of it, but when she was awake there were plenty of offers to hold her and keep her amused. My granddaughter was awake for most of the evening and Darren danced with Lucy while holding her. Emma loved the rotating glitterball hanging from the ceiling and casting a slow-moving pattern of colourful lights over the floor and walls.

As the evening drew to a close Adrian and Kirsty left first, to the cheers and applause of the rest of us. They were booked into the hotel for the night and then going to their flat in the morning. The decorating wasn't finished, but the flat was habitable. Adrian, like Kirsty, had been taking his clothes and other personal possessions there a little at a time. They planned to go on a honeymoon after the schools broke up in July, as Kirsty was a teacher.

I drove home on a high of happiness with Paula dozing in the passenger seat and Darcy-May sound asleep in the back of the car. The arrangements for the day had gone like clockwork, everyone had enjoyed themselves and my son was now married to the lovely Kirsty. It was one of those times when I felt so grateful to be alive. I was on cloud nine, but it wasn't long before reality returned.

* * *

The following day Paula and I slept in and Darcy-May didn't wake for her early-morning bottle until 7 a.m., and then went back to sleep. It was 11 a.m. before I was showered and dressed. I was in the kitchen making myself some breakfast while reading messages on the wedding WhatsApp group. Lots of messages from guests saying how much they had enjoyed the day and sharing their photographs. Having fed Darcy-May, I poured coffee and made buttered toast as she lay in the bouncing cradle, watching me. Paula was still in bed. I heard the letterbox in the front door snap shut as if mail had arrived, but I assumed it was a flyer as there was no mail delivery on Sundays. When I eventually went to see what had been pushed through the letterbox I found not a flyer, but an envelope with my name handwritten in pen on the front.

Puzzled, I opened it as I returned to Darcy-May. I slid out the sheet of paper, which looked as though it had been torn from a school notebook, and read:

Dear Cathy

Thank you for visiting me in hospital and being my foster mum. You are such a nice person. I love you. Can I come and see you soon? I hope you say yes. Call or text me any time you like and I will reply. My number is 07*** ******.
Thank you for being my foster mother. I love you so much.
Haylea xxxxxxx

With the letter still in my hand and leaving Darcy-May in the bouncing cradle, I quickly went out of the front door and looked up and down the street, but Haylea wasn't in sight. I returned indoors and to Darcy-May.

She looked at me from the bouncing cradle. Dear me, I thought. What a letter! Haylea was crying out for love and affection, confirming she'd had very little or none in the past. It was worrying, touching and very needy. However, she wasn't the first child I'd fostered who'd called me Mum and had told me they loved me very early on, but she was the eldest, by far. Younger children I'd looked after, craving warmth and affection and wanting to be liked, had sometimes called me Mummy and said they loved me. But Haylea was fifteen and not my foster child; she barely knew me. It was her obvious desperation to form an attachment that worried me more than the fact she'd been to my house again.

Concerned for Haylea's safety and wellbeing, I took Darcy-May into the living room and phoned Waysbury Children's Home.

'Hello, Dan speaking,' a young man answered.

'It's Cathy Glass, I'm a foster carer. Is Fran, the manager, there?'

'No, it's her day off. Can I help you?'

'Perhaps. Haylea Walsh lives there and has just been to my house and pushed a note through the door.'

'OK,' he said easily. 'I think she said something to her key worker about going to see you. Just a minute, I'll check.'

I waited until he came back on the line.

'Yes, it's OK. She told Dylis she was going to see you,' he said, clearly knowing very little about Haylea's situation.

'I'm fostering her baby and I'm sure she's not supposed to just turn up here. Did someone there clear it with her social worker first?'

'I don't know. I don't suppose so. It's Sunday so the social workers aren't in the office. If you put Haylea on, I'll talk to her.'

'She's not here,' I said, slightly frustrated. 'She just pushed a note through my door about fifteen minutes ago and left.'

'OK.'

It wasn't OK, but I could see I wasn't going to get much from Dan and I could hear voices in the background so I guessed he was busy.

'I take it Haylea isn't back there yet?' I checked.

'No. I don't think so. I haven't seen her.'

'When she arrives can someone let me know she's returned safely, please. And also tell Fran what's happened. I'll tell Haylea's social worker.'

'OK,' he said again.

'Thank you.'

I wasn't convinced I would be told that Haylea had returned and I was worried about her. It was Sunday; Shari wasn't at work so I couldn't speak to her. I knew I could phone the duty social worker for advice in an emergency, but this wasn't an emergency. I just wanted to make sure Haylea was safe. Darcy-May was agitating to be out of the bouncing cradle so I settled her on a blanket on the floor, then texted Haylea.

Hi Haylea. I got your letter. Are you going back to Waysbury now? Cathy x.

Her reply was instant. *Hi Cathy. Thank you for texting. Yes. I'm on the bus now. Can I see you again soon? Love Haylea xx.*

We will need to talk to Shari about that, I replied.

If she says yes can I come to see you again? Please.

My heart went out to her, but I couldn't make promises I might not be able to keep. *Let's see what Shari says first*, I replied. *Have a good day x.*

And you. I love you so much x.

Take care, I replied.

Half an hour later another text arrived from Haylea. *I'm back now. Lots of love Haylea xxxx.*

Thanks for letting me know.

It's nice you care about me xx, she texted back.

Have a good day x, I replied.

I put my phone to one side to concentrate on Darcy-May and all the things I needed to do, but it buzzed with text messages from Haylea for the rest of the day.

Haylea here. What are you doing? I'm in my room watching television …

I love having you as a foster mother. I mean, I know you're not really, but I like to think you are.

I'm still watching television. Love Haylea.

And so it continued. Sometimes I replied but not always. I didn't think I should be encouraging her, so I kept my replies short and reserved, but it didn't stop her texts coming.

I'm going to help Cook now. Speak later. Love you …

Cook says hi. So I guessed Haylea had told Cook she was texting me.

What are you having for your dinner? I'm having pie, mash and peas.

Then later: *I'm in the lounge with some of the others. We're all on our phones.*

At 10.30 I texted: *I'm switching off my phone now as I'm going to bed. Goodnight.*

Nite Nite Cathy. I love you xxxx

Of course I couldn't sleep. Had I done wrong in texting Haylea to check she was safe and on her way back to Waysbury? It seemed to have opened a floodgate. But not once had Haylea mentioned Darcy-May. While her messages showed a vulnerable, needy, unloved young person, there was a positive side. She was reaching out to someone, communicating in a way she hadn't before, and her texts had sounded quite upbeat and positive. She had been in the lounge with other residents, all on their phones, hopefully making friends. I thought the next step would be for her to start talking to someone about what had happened. It's impossible to fully heal if you don't acknowledge and deal with the past, however painful that might be.

Sadly, the following morning the upbeat nature of Haylea's messages had gone. I switched on my phone as soon as I woke and it was flooded with messages from her – text and voice. Waysbury Children's Home couldn't have the same policy as I and most other foster carers had – insisting that phones and other electronic devices are switched off or left downstairs for the night. As I read and listened to the messages, her mood darkened. I grew more and more worried.

I wish you could have been my mother. I never had a proper mummy …

I don't like my life …

I love you but I don't know if you love me …

I wish I'd never been born …

I hate my life …

I've got nothing to live for …

Everyone hates me …

I don't want to wake up in the morning. And so on.

The last one was sent at 4 a.m.: *I want to go to sleep forever.*

My stomach churned. It was 6.20 now. I'd just fed Darcy-May. Was Haylea still awake? I texted: *I've just got your messages. I'm worried about you. Are you all right?*

No reply. I felt sick with fear. She'd sounded desperate, alone in her room at night. Supposing she'd tried to take her own life again and I was the only person she'd contacted. I'd told her I was switching off my phone so she must have known I wouldn't read her messages or reply until the morning – when it could be too late. With my heart racing, I telephoned Waysbury, assuming there was someone on night duty, but it went through to answerphone. I left a message. 'It's Cathy Glass, foster carer. Haylea Walsh has been texting me all night. Can someone check on her, please, and make sure she's all right? She sounded very depressed. I'm worried. Thank you.'

If no one got back to me, I'd phone again shortly. I tried to concentrate on Darcy-May and settled her in the cot so I could get dressed. I took my phone with me into the bathroom in case someone from Waysbury returned my call. They didn't.

I called again and the answerphone cut in. 'It's Cathy Glass,' I said. 'I hope you got my previous message about Haylea. Could someone let me know how she is, please?'

No one called back and, not knowing what to do for the best, I tried phoning again at 8 a.m. To my relief the phone was answered.

'Hello?' said a voice that could have been Fran's.

'It's Cathy Glass. I telephoned earlier and left some messages on your answerphone about Haylea Walsh.'

'Yes, hi, Cathy, it's Fran, the manager. I got your messages. I've just come on duty and I've spoken to Haylea. She said she's sorry she kept texting all night, but she couldn't sleep.'

'She needn't apologize. I was worried. She sounded so down. She needs help.'

'I know. She's been telling Cook she's fed up with her life and wished you could be her mother. I've got a meeting with her social worker today and a member of the mental-health team, so hopefully we can persuade Haylea to see a therapist.'

'Good, thank you. That sounds hopeful.'

CHAPTER ELEVEN

I HATE MY LIFE

I didn't receive any messages from Haylea on that Monday, nor did I hear from Shari, despite having emailed her with an update. Kirsty's mother posted on the wedding WhatsApp group, thanking everyone for coming and for the lovely messages. She included a link to the photographer's website where pictures of the wedding could be viewed online and ordered. Kirsty posted a message on behalf of her and Adrian, thanking everyone for making their day special and for all the presents.

It was Tuesday afternoon before Shari telephoned. She began as she usually did by thanking me for my email. 'How is Darcy-May?' she asked. It was easy to forget that Darcy-May was the child I was fostering with everything going on around Haylea.

'Absolutely fine,' I said. 'I take her to the clinic each week to be weighed and measured. She's putting on weight and developing as she should. Her Red Book is up to date. I'm taking lots of photographs and have begun her Life Story Book.'

'Thank you. I'm expecting an update from the permanency team soon. And I had a meeting yesterday at Waysbury. Haylea has agreed to see a therapist.'

'Excellent,' I said.

'She has also asked if she could see you. Once a week for a couple of hours. We think it's probably a good idea.'

'Oh, OK,' I said tentatively. 'Where?'

'She would like to come to your house.'

'You know Darcy-May will be here? I can't hide her away.'

'We don't foresee a problem. Haylea was offered contact and if she'd accepted it she would be seeing Darcy-May at least once a week until she went for adoption.'

'You don't think she'll start to bond with Darcy-May, making it more painful when she has to say goodbye?' I asked. But even as I said it I thought that was highly unlikely from what I'd seen so far.

'Haylea understands Darcy-May will be with you, but she said she will ignore her.'

'Which is what she has been doing – at contact and when she came here.'

'Yes, I know, I saw that in the report. So I'll tell Haylea she can come to see you once a week for a couple of hours. Is any day better for you than another? While Haylea isn't in school she can do any day. She has suggested Wednesday.'

'All right. So, starting tomorrow?'

'Yes.'

'And what about text messages?'

'Yes, if that's all right with you.'

'As long as Haylea understands that if I'm busy I won't be able to reply straight away, and that my phone is switched off at night. I was very worried when I turned it on in the morning to find all those desperate messages.'

104

'We talked about that yesterday. Haylea knows she should have gone to the care worker on night duty if she was upset.'

'OK.'

'And please include Haylea's visits when you complete your weekly report on Darcy-May,' Shari said. 'I'll let Joy know what we've agreed.' Suddenly the arrangement for Haylea seeing me appeared more formal. 'Obviously if she discloses abuse or anything else we should know, you'll tell us.'

'Yes, of course.' It's part of the foster carer's role to pass on information affecting the child to their social worker.

An hour later – the time it took Shari to phone Haylea – she texted me.

Shari just called and I can visit you every week for ever! I'm so pleased you can be my foster mum. Thank you. I love you so much xxx

I felt sure Shari hadn't phrased it that way, and of course Haylea's reaction was over the top, but Shari, and presumably the other professionals who'd agreed to Haylea being in contact with me, knew the tone of her messages. Nevertheless, I would keep all her messages as well as making notes on our meeting, just in case they were needed in the future, and to cover myself.

See you tomorrow, I replied to Haylea.

She texted straight back: *I'm looking forward to it so much. Love you loads xxx.*

Haylea sent six more texts that day telling me what she was doing and that she was looking forward to seeing me tomorrow. There was also a voice message, and her excitement at seeing me was palpable. I replied by text, not voicemail, low key and confirming I'd see her at 2 p.m. the next day. There were no messages that night but plenty the following morning: telling me what she was having for breakfast, that she was looking forward to seeing me, and she'd be leaving soon to get on the bus. She then texted to say she would be early, which I'd guessed from the time she left the house.

However, when she arrived – at 1.30 – her euphoria had gone and her mood had changed.

I answered the door and could see straight away she was down.

'What's the matter?' I asked as she came into the hall.

She shrugged. We went into the living room where I offered her a drink, but she didn't want one. Darcy-May was upstairs in her cot having an afternoon sleep. The baby monitor was on. Haylea sat on the sofa, head hung low. She was wearing a below-the-knee floral dress, similar to the others I'd seen her wearing before, with a long cardigan.

'What's the matter?' I asked again as I sat in one of the chairs.

She shrugged. 'I can't tell you.'

'Have you told someone at Waysbury or your social worker?'

She shook her head.

'You sounded very positive in your messages. What has changed?'

'I've got to see a doctor,' she said gloomily.

'Are you ill?'

'I don't know.'

'Is something hurting?'

'No.'

'Do you feel unwell?'

'No.'

'So what makes you think you need to see a doctor?' I asked.

She couldn't look at me.

'Someone at the hospital phoned and said I should go.'

'You've been to the hospital?'

'When I had the baby.'

This wasn't making any sense. 'Do you need treatment?' I asked.

'I think so.'

'Haylea, love, I really don't understand. I can't help you if you don't tell me what the problem is.'

'If I tell you, you'll think I'm a dirty slut.'

'Of course I won't.' And for a moment I wondered if she was pregnant again. 'I've fostered a lot of young people, as well as bringing up three children of my own,' I said. 'I know the problems that can arise, sometimes very personal problems.'

Haylea hesitated, kept her gaze away from me and chewed her bottom lip. 'The hospital did some tests when I had the baby,' she said at last. 'I had an infection. They gave me antibiotics and want me to go back to check the infection's all gone.'

'That sounds like normal practice to me, so what's the problem?'

'They have to take a swab – you know, down there. It freaked me out last time. I'm not going again.'

'Do you have an STI – a sexually transmitted infection?' I asked matter-of-factly.

'Yes. I told you I was a slut.'

'Of course you're not,' I said firmly. 'And please don't call yourself that. You're not the first young person I've

107

known who has contracted an STI, but it is important you go back for a follow-up appointment to make sure the infection has completely gone. Otherwise it can come back and cause long-term health problems, including damaging other parts of your body and some cancers.'

'That's what the nurse said, but if I go back they're going to take another swab and ask me who I slept with. I can't tell them.'

'They need to trace the person so they can be treated too,' I said. 'Otherwise they will continue to spread the infection to others.'

'I can't tell them, he'd kill me,' she said, her face contorting with anguish.

'You mean the baby's father?' I asked.

She nodded. I would have liked to give her a hug if I'd felt she wanted one. Instead, I left my chair and sat beside her on the sofa.

'Haylea, love. I understand why you're worried, but he wouldn't be told who had given his name. He will be contacted and asked to go for a test, that's all. They won't say you told them. He probably doesn't know he has an infection and could be spreading it to others.' I felt sad I was having this conversation with a fifteen-year-old, but it had to be said.

'I don't have his details so I can't tell them,' Haylea said. 'I mean, I know what he looks like, but I don't know where he lives.'

'So you don't still see him?'

She shook her head. 'It wasn't like that.'

'All right. Tell the nurse what you know, but it's still important you go back for your follow-up appointment to make sure the infection has completely gone.'

Haylea gave a small nod.

'And you haven't told Shari or anyone at Waysbury about this?' I asked.

'No.'

'We need to. Then someone can go with you.'

'Will you come with me?' she asked.

'I can't really, love. I'm looking after Darcy-May. But I'm sure someone from Waysbury can go with you. Perhaps your key worker, Dylis?'

'Can you tell them?'

'If that's what you want.'

'Yes.'

Darcy-May could now be heard through the monitor, gurgling as she woke. 'I'll need to fetch her,' I said.

'If I go now will you phone Fran so she knows by the time I get back?' Haylea asked.

'Yes, love. But there's nothing to be embarrassed about. I'm sure Fran and Shari will have dealt with this before.'

She looked at me, haunted and scared.

'Don't worry, I'll talk to them.'

She was eager to go now, so I saw her to the door. Then I went upstairs, changed Darcy-May and brought her down, where I gave her a bottle before I phoned Waysbury.

Fran answered. 'It's Cathy Glass. Haylea left me about fifteen minutes ago. She's on her way back, but she asked me to call you. She's embarrassed because she has an STI. It seems she was tested when she was in hospital having her baby. She was prescribed antibiotics and has been asked to go back for a follow-up appointment to check the infection has gone. She doesn't want to go because she's worried about having another swab taken and also that they will ask her for details of her sexual partners. I've reassured her as best I could, but can someone there talk to her and go with her?'

'Yes, of course. Poor girl. She should have told us. Does her social worker know?'

'I don't think so. Haylea hasn't told her.'

'Probably not then. At Haylea's age she is entitled to the same confidentiality in these matters as an adult.' Which I knew from my foster-carer training. As long as the practitioner is satisfied that the young person is capable of understanding the information and decisions involved, then the parent, carer or guardian would not automatically be told.

'Haylea said she couldn't give the details of the baby's father as he'd kill her if he found out, to use her words.'

'Sounds like a nice person,' Fran said grimly.

'That's what I thought. Haylea said she doesn't see him any more.'

'All right. I'll talk with her when she gets back. Dylis can book the appointment and go with her.'

'Good. I'll see Haylea again next Wednesday then.'

We said goodbye and about ten minutes later Haylea texted.

I'm nearly there. Have you told them?

Yes, I replied. *I spoke to Fran. It's fine. Don't worry. She'll see you when you get back.*

What did she say? Is she angry with me? Haylea texted.

No. Of course not. She understands and will help you. Dylis should be able to go with you to the appointment.

I'm scared.

Don't be. It'll be fine.

An hour later Haylea texted to say she'd seen Fran

and *she was so nice and kind. Everyone is kind to me. I don't deserve it.*

Of course you deserve it, I replied. *You're a nice person. Have a good evening.*

Later Haylea texted that she was helping Cook and seemed in a better mood. But at 9 p.m. she messaged: *I hate my life.*

Are you alone in your room? I asked.

Yes.

Please go and talk to someone. Don't sit there all by yourself and get down.

I can't talk to anyone. They would hate me if they knew.

I am sure they wouldn't. Know what?

Nothing.

When are you seeing the therapist? I asked.

Friday.

Please don't be alone. Is there anyone in the lounge you can be with?

I don't know.

I didn't hear any more from Haylea and I was worried she could be alone in her room growing more and more depressed. Yet I felt I shouldn't encourage a dependency on me by texting repeatedly to ask if she was all right. She had her social worker and the team at Waysbury, and she was seeing her therapist soon. But it didn't stop me worrying about her. Had she been my foster child I would have known her better, able to judge her mood and on hand to offer support as necessary. As it was, I imagined all sorts of outcomes. At 10.30, as I was getting ready for bed, I texted: *Are you OK?*

It was half an hour before she replied. *I'm OK. Thanks for caring about me.*

Lots of people care about you, I texted back. *I hope you have a good night's sleep. I'm going to sleep now so I'll turn off my phone. Good night.*

She must have slept late the following morning for she didn't text again until lunchtime: *I'm sorry for being such a pain. You must be fed up with me.*

I am not fed up with you, I replied. *But I am worried about you.*

That's nice. No one has ever worried about me before.

Which I thought could be true.

Haylea continued to text every so often throughout the day and for the rest of the week, often about what she was doing or not doing – *I'm bored, everyone is out … I've got to go out for a walk now … I'm in my room … I'm having dinner … I'm fed up …* and so forth. Her mood always dipped at night when she was alone in her room. I encouraged her to talk to whoever was on duty. Whether she did or not, I didn't know. Perhaps the staff assumed she was asleep. I noted it all when I wrote up my log notes for Darcy-May as Shari had asked me to.

On Friday morning Haylea texted: *I'm going to see the therapist soon xx.*

Good luck x.

I was hoping that talking to the therapist would set Haylea on the path to recovery, although I knew that counselling or therapy didn't suit everyone. The time has to be right and the client must feel they can engage with the therapist so they are free to explore their innermost pain and fears. Haylea had agreed to go, so I was hopeful it would prove useful.

I was wrong.

CHAPTER TWELVE

SPARE BEDROOM

You're going to hate me, Haylea's text message read.

It was 1 p.m. on Friday afternoon and I knew she must have recently come out of her first counselling session. I was getting ready to see Lucy and my granddaughter. It was a sunny day and we planned to go to a park near where Lucy lived. Leaving the house with a baby is never instant and I was checking the baby bag to make sure I had everything I needed. Darcy-May was in the bouncing cradle, grinning at me. I stopped what I was doing to reply to Haylea's text.

I'm not going to hate you. What's the matter? Did you see the therapist? I wondered if perhaps she hadn't gone.

I went.

What's the matter then?

I didn't talk to her.

Don't worry. I expect she's used to that. You may feel like talking to her next time.

I should have talked to her. It was bad of me not to. I'm an evil person.

No, you're not x.

You don't know what I've done. You'd hate me if you knew.

A frisson of fear ran through me. I sat on the sofa and looked at Darcy-May.

What is it I should know, Haylea? I texted back. *I'm sure it's not that bad.* I wondered if I should phone her, but her next text arrived immediately.

It is very bad.

Have you told anyone?

No. I can't.

Can you tell me?

I hate my life. I want to die.

I phoned her, but she didn't answer. I waited, tried again and then texted Lucy to say I was going to be late. Still nothing from Haylea, so I texted her again: *Are you at Waysbury? If so, please talk to someone there.*

I can't, came her reply.

Then tell me what's wrong.

No text message, but then my phone began to ring and Haylea's number showed on the caller display. I quickly answered.

'Hello, love,' I said gently. The only sound was her crying. 'Haylea, what's the matter? Where are you?' I waited. She continued to cry. 'Haylea, please talk to me.'

'Oh Cathy, I wish I was dead.'

'No. Nothing is so bad that it can't be fixed.'

'This is.'

'What, love?'

Silence, then, 'Can I ask you something?'

'Yes, of course.' Darcy-May had stopped grinning and was now looking at me seriously, as if sensing her mother's distress. 'What is it, love?' I asked Haylea.

More silence and then, 'If you knew someone was being hurt and you didn't tell because you were scared of what might happen to you, does that make you a bad person?'

I tried to unravel what she was telling me.

'It wouldn't make you a bad person, but if I knew someone was being hurt, I would do all I could to help them and stop it from happening again, including telling someone. Haylea, do you know someone who is being hurt?'

Silence.

'Haylea?'

'Yes,' she said quietly.

'Who?'

She didn't reply.

'Haylea, who is being hurt?'

'Others like me.'

'Like you? You mean another young person?'

'Yes.' I went cold.

'Who?'

'I can't tell you.'

'Where do they live?'

Silence.

'Haylea? Where does this person live?'

'Perhaps it's stopped now,' she said.

'Haylea, if you know or suspect that a child or young person is being hurt or has been hurt, then you need to tell someone. If not me, then your social worker, someone at Waysbury, or the police.'

'No, I can't!' she cried, and cut the call.

I tried phoning back, but she didn't answer. I texted: *Haylea, please answer your phone. I need to talk to you.*

She didn't, so I telephoned Waysbury. 'Is Fran there, please?'

'No. Who's speaking?'

'Cathy Glass.'

'Hi, Cathy, it's Dylis, Haylea's key worker.'

'Is Haylea there?'

'No, I dropped her off in the town after counselling this morning. Why?'

'She just called me, very upset.' I then told Dylis what Haylea had said about someone being hurt and not telling.

'Oh dear, that doesn't sound good,' Dylis said. 'I'll phone her.'

'She said she couldn't talk to the therapist this morning.'

'I don't know what was said. I waited outside the room. She was in there for nearly an hour. She has another appointment next week.'

'Was she upset when she left?'

'No. Just quiet. But then Haylea is often quiet. We do what we can to draw her out and include her.'

'Perhaps something happened after she left you?' I suggested.

'I'll phone her now,' Dylis said.

'Thank you.'

There wasn't anything else I could do, so I texted Lucy to say I was on my way and left with Darcy-May in the car seat, the baby bag over my shoulder and deep in thought. In truth, Haylea hadn't really said much, but it was the way she'd said it – the suggestion she knew someone was being hurt or had been, set against the backdrop of how she was – a very troubled young person. It was possible Haylea was exaggerating, jumping to conclusions or even making it up, but a gut feeling from years of fostering told me she wasn't. I hoped Dylis would have more success in encouraging Haylea to share the details of what she knew. Haylea's comment about her being evil was playing on my mind too.

It was nice seeing Lucy and Emma again, but if I'm honest thoughts of Haylea clouded the afternoon. I didn't tell Lucy and worry her. If Haylea was right and a child was being abused then it was possible it was still happening, right now, at this very moment. It was a harrowing thought and one I kept returning to during the afternoon. I checked my phone regularly, but there was nothing from Haylea. I doubted I'd get any feedback from Dylis, as I wasn't fostering Haylea.

Emma, nearly eleven months old, enjoyed being pushed on the swings and then sitting on Lucy's lap to come down the slide or go on the roundabout. She was able to toddle while holding her mother's hand. Darcy-May, at three months, was too young to join in yet, but enjoyed watching.

It was 4 p.m. when we left the park. I walked with Lucy back to her flat where I'd left my car and then drove home. I fell into what had become my evening routine – seeing to Darcy-May and preparing dinner for Paula and me. The dinner table seemed rather empty now Adrian and Lucy had gone and I wasn't fostering an older child. I couldn't remember the last time there had just been the two of us, night after night.

Later that evening, when I typed up my log notes, I included Haylea's text messages and phone call. I also emailed Shari the details and copied in Joy. It was up to Shari now what she did with the information. On a more positive note, Adrian telephoned and invited us for dinner on Sunday.

The following Wednesday Darcy-May had an appointment at the clinic for her second dose of the six-in-one vaccine. As before, I was dreading it and she cried as the needle stabbed her arm, but she soon recovered. It was a month before the next one.

I hadn't heard any more from Haylea and I was wondering if she was still coming to see me that afternoon. When it got to 2.30 and she hadn't arrived I texted her: *Are you coming today?* If she wasn't, I could get on with something else.

Haylea didn't reply and I wondered if perhaps she was able to talk to Dylis now so didn't need me. However, I was still concerned for her, so half an hour later, when she still hadn't replied, I texted again: *Are you OK?*

It was another thirty minutes before she replied, and when I read her message my heart sank. *Someone is being hurt but I can't tell anyone.*

Was this for real? I wondered. Or was she playing with my feelings?

I tried phoning her, but she didn't answer, so I texted: *You need to tell someone. Is Dylis there?*

No, she replied straight away.

What about Fran or another care worker?

I can't tell them. Can you tell someone for me?

I can, I replied. *But I will need to tell them where the information came from. Who is being hurt?*

A few minutes passed and then another text arrived. *They may be at* – She gave an address that I knew was about three miles away on the other side of town.

Who is there? I texted back.

A brother and sister.

And you think they are being hurt?

Yes.

I needed to talk to Haylea and I tried phoning but she didn't answer. I really didn't know what to believe.

What are their names? I texted.

I'm not sure. My doubts increased.

How old are they?

About five and seven I think.

How do you know they are being hurt?

Another pause and then, *I just do.*

And that was it. No more messages. I tried phoning again, but she didn't answer, so I wondered again if Haylea was toying with me for whatever reason. But I couldn't take the risk. I phoned Waysbury and asked for Fran or Dylis, but neither of them was available. I then explained to the care worker I was speaking to who I was and that Haylea Walsh had been texting me, saying she knew two children were being abused and had sent me an address, but that was all.

'She's in the house somewhere,' the care worker said. 'I'll go and find her and talk to her.'

'Thank you.'

I then phoned Shari and repeated what Haylea had told me.

'What address did she give?' Shari asked.

I read it out as she wrote it down.

'And she didn't tell you their names?'

'No.'

'How does Haylea know these children?' Shari asked.

'I don't know. She wouldn't say any more.'

'I'll speak to her.'

At that point I still had doubts about the truthfulness of what Haylea was claiming. It was so vague. There was a chance she was attention-seeking – craving the love, care and affection she hadn't received as a child. It does happen that a child or young person makes a false allegation, and it can ruin lives. Although usually it's about themselves being abused, not someone else.

The following day Joy telephoned to arrange her next visit, unaware of this latest development. I told her and read out Haylea's text messages. She said she'd ask Shari what action was being taken and would let me know.

Haylea texted the following day: *Did the police go to that address?*

I don't know. Were the police informed?

They came to see me.

I don't know any more. You will need to ask Shari. Well done for talking to the police. Are you all right?

I'm scared.

I tried phoning her but she didn't answer, so I texted: *What can I do to help?*

Nothing. No one can help me.

Yes, lots of people want to help you. Are you at Waysbury?

Yes.

Can you talk to Dylis?

No. Thank you for caring.

And that was it. No more texts and she didn't answer her phone. This was playing havoc with my feelings and I was worried for Haylea. The fact she'd talked to the police seemed to add credibility to her claims. That evening I emailed Shari saying Haylea was scared and also updated my log notes. It was only when Joy came the following week that I learnt what had happened.

'The police went to the address Haylea gave,' Joy said. 'But no children live there. It's just a single man and he doesn't have children. The police tried to get some more details from Haylea, but she said she didn't know any more. Without the children's names or more details of the alleged abuse there is nothing more they can do.'

Joy asked to see the text messages from Haylea and I gave her my phone. 'I don't think there is any more that can be done at present,' she sighed as she finished reading, and handed it back.

We then began discussing Darcy-May – the main reason for Joy's visit. I showed her the Red Book and we talked about Darcy-May's routine and general development. Joy said there was no further news from the permanency team and ended her visit by looking around the house, especially where Darcy-May slept in my room. Satisfied, she returned downstairs. As we went into the living room for Joy to collect her briefcase I asked, 'The man who lives at the address Haylea gave, does he have a criminal record?'

'I don't know. But I'm sure the police would have checked that. They asked Haylea if it was possible she'd made a mistake with the address and she wouldn't answer.'

'Do you think she could be making it up?' I asked her.

'I think she could be very confused.'

'I am worried about her,' I said.

'I know.'

I saw Joy out and then concentrated on Darcy-May. She was now having 'tummy time' each day. This involved placing her on her front on a blanket on the floor so she could kick, twist and move her limbs. It helped strengthen neck muscles and develop limb coordination, which would eventually lead to crawling. In line with current practice, I was doing it a few times each day. Darcy-May enjoyed it, for a short time at least, and then wanted to be picked up.

Two days later Joy telephoned and when she said, 'Cathy, you've got a spare bedroom, and you're approved to foster teenagers,' I thought I knew what she was going to say, but I was wrong. There is always a shortage of foster carers, not everyone is approved to foster teenagers and I had a spare bedroom.

'That's right,' I replied. 'But I'm happy just looking after Darcy-May at present.'

'Yes, I can see that, and you're doing a good job. But I've just had a long chat with Shari. She's asking if you can take Haylea.'

'What?' I exclaimed. 'As well as her baby?'

'Yes. Shari thinks Haylea would do better in a foster placement and Haylea is asking to come to you.'

All manner of concerns flashed through my mind. 'But what about Darcy-May?' I said. 'Haylea will be living with her, seeing her every day. They will bond.'

'We discussed that, but most mothers who are being assessed have their babies with them to begin with, even if they can't keep them.' Which I knew, but we seemed to be seeing this very differently. Why risk creating a bond which would have to be broken if there was no need? 'Haylea is asking to come to you,' Joy said. 'She feels you are the only person she can talk to.'

'I don't know,' I said. 'Can't she talk to her therapist?'

'She's attending the sessions, but she hasn't talked to her yet.'

That wasn't helping my decision. 'Shari told me that Haylea's family has had involvement with the social services. What was all that about?' As I was being asked to foster Haylea I had a right to know.

'It was when Haylea's mother left and her father had a new partner. A neighbour phoned the police with concerns and felt Haylea was being neglected. She said she'd been worried before the mother had left but hadn't said anything. A social worker – not Shari – visited the family twice. The father and stepmother were looking after Haylea and seemed to be putting her needs first. Haylea appeared reasonably well cared for, although she didn't have much of a routine. At the follow-up visit it was noted that changes had been made and the concerns had largely gone. I can send you the placement information form if you wish.'

'Yes, please. Has Haylea been in trouble with the police at all?' I asked. 'I know her father has a criminal record and her brother is in prison now.'

'No. Never. She's introverted and lacks confidence but should thrive in a foster placement. She's struggling to fit in at Waysbury.'

'Yes, I know. What about school?' I asked.

'She is being found a new one and in the meantime we will arrange for a home tutor to visit her for a few sessions a week.'

I paused to think. 'If I say yes, how long will Haylea be with me?'

'Until she's eighteen and leaves care.'

'So, after Darcy-May goes for adoption?'

'Yes, that's the care plan.'

'What will happen if I don't agree to take her?'

'She'll be found another carer, but Haylea wants you.'

'Can I think about it?' I asked.

'Yes. I'll phone you tomorrow.'

Not only did I need to think about taking Haylea, but I needed to discuss it with Paula too. Sometimes children just arrived at very short notice in an emergency, but if it was a planned moved, as this was, then I liked to discuss it with my family first. Not Adrian or Lucy any more; they no longer lived at home, so fostering Haylea wasn't going to have the same impact on their lives as it would on Paula's. I would tell them if and when Haylea came to live with us.

Paula agreed, and the following day Haylea moved in.

CHAPTER THIRTEEN

TOO GRATEFUL

Joy telephoned me at ten that morning for my decision and Haylea arrived at 4 p.m. Shari brought her, with two very large storage-style bags containing her belongings.

'Thank you for being my foster mother,' Haylea said as soon as I opened the door. Coming in, she threw her arms around me and gave me a hug. I was taken aback. She'd shied away from physical contact before and I couldn't remember ever having such a warm welcome from a child or young person who'd just arrived. Usually they were upset, angry and resentful at having to leave home or their previous foster placement.

'That's a good beginning,' Shari said, also coming in.

'We're in the living room,' I said.

Leaving the bags in the hall for unpacking later, I led the way down the hall and into the living room. Darcy-May was in the bouncing cradle by the chair I'd just vacated.

'Hi, gorgeous,' Shari said, making a fuss of her.

I automatically glanced at Haylea to see if she would react, but there was nothing. She didn't give Darcy-May a second look and, sitting on the sofa, gazed towards the patio doors. It was lovely and warm outside and the doors were slightly open. Sammy could be seen lying on the patio in the shade.

'They gave me a leaving present,' Haylea said, bringing her attention back and referring to the jeweller's box she was holding. 'It's a necklace.' She lifted the lid to show me.

'That's lovely,' I said.

'They gave me a good luck card too. It's in one of the bags in the hall.'

'Great. We can stand it on a shelf in your bedroom later when we unpack.'

Shari had taken her laptop from her briefcase and was waiting for it to load so she could complete the necessary forms for placing a child. I sat in the chair by Darcy-May.

'Joy emailed you the placement information?' Shari asked me.

'Yes, thank you.'

'She's hoping to join us.'

I nodded. Ideally the carer's supervising social worker is present when a child is placed, but that's not always possible.

'A lot of this I already know because you are fostering Darcy-May,' Shari said, looking at a file on her laptop. 'I can fill that in later. Is it just you and Paula here now?' she asked.

'Yes.'

'And the cat,' Haylea said, as a much younger child might.

'That's right.' I smiled.

The doorbell rang and I went to answer it. It was Joy.

'Sorry I'm late. I got held up,' she said. 'Are they here?'

'They've just arrived.'

She came with me into the living room where I introduced her to Haylea and then offered everyone a drink.

'Just a glass of water, please,' Joy said. No one else wanted anything.

'Shall I help you?' Haylea offered.

'No, love, it's OK, thanks.'

As I left the living room Joy was making a fuss of Darcy-May, but then she began to grizzle, either because she'd had enough of being in the bouncing cradle or all the new faces in the room.

'Shall I pick her up?' Joy called as I poured her a glass of water.

'Yes, please.'

I returned to the living room and placed the glass of water within Joy's reach. Darcy-May was still grizzling so Joy passed her to me. Haylea appeared oblivious to Darcy-May's upset. I saw Shari watching her for a reaction too.

Joy took out a notepad and pen. Darcy-May settled on my lap and Shari began going through the routine for placing a child. She checked with Haylea that she wasn't taking any medication – she'd finished the course of antibiotics.

'Are there any more follow-up appointments at the hospital?' I asked.

'No. Haylea has been given the all-clear,' Shari said. She continued to say that Haylea didn't have any allergies or special dietary requirements, and told me how much allowance Haylea was entitled to at her age. I said I would give it to her every Saturday.

'Does Haylea have a savings account yet?' Joy asked. When a child first comes into care it's usual to open a savings account for them and add to it each week.

'Not yet,' Shari replied, glancing up from typing. 'They didn't have a chance to do it at Waysbury.'

'I'll open one,' I said. 'And how much am I putting on her mobile phone?' I asked. Sometimes this can be an issue if the young person uses their phone a lot.

'You've hardly been using any credit, have you?' Shari asked Haylea.

'No. I've still got plenty.'

'We'll top it up as and when you need it then,' I said.

Shari and Joy both made a note. If a young person consistently runs out of credit then they are expected to budget so it lasts.

'Do you like your phone?' Joy asked Haylea, aware that she hadn't had one before going to Waysbury.

'Yes, I've got more phone numbers now,' she replied proudly. 'Some of those at Waysbury gave me theirs before I left. They are going to text me.'

'That's good,' Joy replied, and threw her a knowing smile. Haylea's reply and her manner were quaint, as though she wasn't used to any of this.

'Haylea's toiletries and beauty products?' Shari asked. 'Will she be expected to pay for them from her allowance or will they come out of your weekly household shop?'

'I'll buy them,' I said. 'Haylea can come with me and choose what she wants.' If a young person is expected to buy these items then they are given more in their allowance.

'I don't have beauty products,' Haylea said. 'I'm not beautiful.'

'Of course you're beautiful,' I said. 'And you don't need products to make you beautiful. It's the person within.'

'Exactly,' Joy agreed.

'Cathy will buy you what you need,' Shari clarified, as if talking to a younger child. 'Including toiletries, sanitary towels and anything else you need. Just tell her.'

'Thank you,' Haylea said. 'You're all so kind to me. I like it here.'

Again, I could tell from Joy's expression that she was struggling with what to make of Haylea, as I had when I'd first met her. She had the manner, attitude and appearance of a much older woman, but it was as though there was a small child inside. Not at all like the average teenager.

'Can you register Haylea with your doctor?' Shari asked. It was usual for the looked-after child to be registered with the foster carer's family doctor.

'Yes, it will be the same one you have on file for Darcy-May.'

'Perfect,' Shari said as she typed.

Shari then gave me details of Haylea's counselling appointments, at present once a week. I offered to take her in my car, but Haylea said she didn't want to be any trouble and could go on the bus.

'It's no trouble,' I said.

'Cathy is here to help you,' Joy said.

Haylea looked unsure what to do. 'I'll leave it up to the two of you to decide,' Shari said, and I nodded.

Once Shari had finished the form-filling, she asked me to sign the form online, in which I agreed to foster Haylea in line with current guidelines. Shari closed her laptop and said she'd have a look around the house before she left. Darcy-May had fallen asleep in my arms so I left the three of them to start looking around the downstairs while I settled her in the cot in my bedroom. Although Haylea had been in my house before, she hadn't seen all the rooms. I heard Joy, who knew my house well from all her visits, giving a guided tour. 'This is the living room where you can watch television ...' and so forth.

I returned downstairs and went into the kitchen-diner where they were.

'Haylea was wondering if she will be able to help with the cooking like she did at Waysbury,' Shari asked me.

'Yes, of course. I'm always pleased to have some help.' I smiled at Haylea.

'But you will be cooking the family meals?' Shari checked. 'Haylea's not expected to cook her own meals?'

'No. We usually eat there,' I said, pointing to the table. 'It will be nice having someone else. There's just been Paula and me recently, although my family come to dinner and lunch sometimes and we go to theirs.'

'And Haylea will come with you when you visit your family?' Shari checked.

'Yes, of course, assuming she wants to. She is part of the family while she is with us.'

I hadn't realized the effect my words would have on Haylea until she sniffed and, with tears in her eyes, said, 'Thank you, Cathy, you're so kind to me. A family.' Her voice broke.

Joy glanced at me as she passed Haylea a tissue from the box I kept in the kitchen. I think Joy thought, as I did, that either Haylea had been completely starved of affection or she was trying to gain my sympathy. Either way, it was both worrying and touching.

Once Haylea had recovered, we continued the tour by going into the front room, and then upstairs. I took them first to Haylea's bedroom and we all went in.

'It will look better once you have your things in here and make it yours,' I said. It was decorated in a neutral colour so it would suit most ages and tastes. As Shari admired the view from the window – this room was at the back of the house and overlooked the garden – Haylea's gaze went to the bedroom door.

'Is there a lock on the door?' she asked me.

'No, love, none of the bedroom doors have locks,' I replied. 'It's not considered safe. Did you have a lock on your bedroom door at home?'

She shook her head.

'No one will come into your bedroom without your permission,' I said. 'It's a house rule. We don't go into each other's bedrooms. If I want you, I will knock first, and I expect you to do the same.' Haylea didn't look convinced.

'There is just Cathy and her daughter Paula living here,' Joy said, seeing Haylea's unease.

'You will meet Paula later,' I added. 'She's twenty-four and is looking forward to meeting you.'

'Is there a lock on the bathroom door?' Shari asked.

'Yes, although it can be opened from the outside in an emergency.' Which was normal practice.

'The same at Waysbury, all the doors can be opened from the outside if necessary,' Shari said. 'Do you have any more questions?' she asked Haylea.

'No, I'm sorry for being a pain.'

'You're not a pain, love,' I said. 'It's important you ask questions.' I went to touch her arm to reassure her, but she moved away, which was interesting. She'd initiated physical contact when she'd first arrived by hugging me, but now didn't like it when I tried to touch her.

We filed out of Haylea's bedroom and round the landing. I pointed out Paula's room, and then continued to my room where Darcy-May was asleep in the cot. Shari and Joy went in quietly while Haylea waited on the landing with me.

'If you need anything in the night, just call me and I'll come to you,' I said, keeping my voice low so I didn't wake Darcy-May. 'I leave a night light on the landing, but I don't want you wandering around by yourself in case you trip and fall. You may hear me get up to feed and change Darcy-May, but I'm as quiet as I can be. Paula doesn't usually hear me.'

'Do you have to get up every night to see to her?' Haylea asked.

'Yes, love,' I replied, and then realized Haylea had asked about Darcy-May. I couldn't remember her ever doing that before; she'd barely acknowledged her existence.

'I'm often awake at night,' Haylea added, which I knew from when she'd texted me during the night at Waysbury.

'Why don't you sleep well?' I asked.

She was about to reply when Joy and Shari came out of my bedroom.

'Thank you,' Shari said, and we went downstairs.

Shari checked with Haylea that she had everything she needed and then she and Joy left. Haylea came with me to see them off at the door.

'Thank you for letting me live with you,' she said as soon as they'd gone.

'I'm pleased to have you,' I replied. 'It's bound to be a bit strange to begin with, but you'll soon get used to it. Ask me if you need anything.'

'I will. Thank you.' She stayed where she was, looking at me awkwardly.

'It's gone five o'clock,' I said. 'I need to get some dinner going for later.'

'I can help you.'

'Or you could start to unpack your belongings,' I suggested, glancing at the two large bags in the hall. 'You'll feel more settled and at home once you have your things around you.'

'Yes, I can start unpacking my belongings,' she replied in her old-fashioned way, repeating what I'd said.

'Great. I'll help you upstairs with the bags.'

We took one each and heaved them up the stairs and into her bedroom. I pointed out the wardrobe, drawers and shelves where her belongings would go. 'I'll be in the kitchen if you want me,' I said. 'What you don't get done now I can help you with later.'

'Thank you, Cathy. Thank you for everything.'

'You're welcome.' I smiled and came out.

I'd just got to the bottom of the stairs when I heard Darcy-May wake. She was due for a feed so I returned upstairs, changed her and then brought her down to feed her. Once she was content, I parked her in the bouncing cradle in the kitchen while I prepared the vegetables for the pasta bake I was making for dinner. As usual I talked to her as I worked – 'This is carrot, yummy, I'm slicing it,' and so on. She often made noises as though she was replying. It was cute and, of course, that's how infants learn language – by hearing it repeated over and over again. I always had her with me in the same room and it was something Haylea was going to have to get used to. Again, I wondered what effect living together would have on Haylea and Darcy-May. Probably little if Haylea had nothing to do with her. As I was Darcy-May's main care-giver she was bonding with me, and if Haylea continued to ignore her then there was no reason for that to change, unless Haylea began engaging with Darcy-May. Supposing she changed her mind about Darcy-May going for adoption? I wondered. Would she stand any chance of being able to keep her baby?

Twenty minutes later, as I put the bake into the oven, I heard Haylea come downstairs.

'In here, love!' I called.

She came into the kitchen. For safety, I'd positioned Darcy May's bouncing cradle where the kitchen met the dining area, away from the cooker and where I was working. Haylea had to step around her to come in but didn't acknowledge her.

'I've unpacked,' she said.

'That was quick. Well done.'

'Would you like to see my room? I've made it nice.' She clearly wanted to show me.

'Yes.'

I took Darcy-May from the bouncing cradle and followed Haylea upstairs. Her room was neat and tidy and she'd packed away all her belongings. She'd arranged cards on the bookshelf – not only her leaving card from Waysbury, but also her birthday cards, which had meant so much to her.

'I know it's not my birthday,' she said, seeing me looking. 'But I can still have my cards out, can't I?'

'Yes, of course, love.' As well as the birthday card I'd given to her, there were three others.

'Who are they from?' I asked.

'This one is from all the staff at Waysbury,' she said, going over and touching it. 'This one is from the other kids who live there. That one is from Shari.'

I nodded. 'So your family didn't send one?' Sometimes they arrived late, having come through the social services.

'No. I don't think they know where I am.'

I nodded. Even so, I knew of other parents with children in care who weren't told where they were but had taken presents and cards to the social services for the social worker to pass on.

'Mum used to give me a card when she lived with us, but I think she's forgotten me now.'

'What about your sister and brothers, are they not in contact?' I asked. According to the placement information form they weren't, but sometimes that can be out of date.

'No.'

'And your father? Did he give you a card and present when you were at home?'

'Yes, but I didn't like his presents. I don't want them any more,' she replied, her face clouding over.

'OK. I just wondered. You've done well unpacking.'

'Thank you. What shall I do with the empty bags?'

'I'll put them away, as you won't need them for a long time.'

'A very long time. Thank you, Cathy. Thank you for having me.'

'You're welcome.' But I heard alarm bells ringing. Never before had I fostered a child who was so grateful to have left home and be with me. Even the most neglected and abused child had some loyalty and longing for home, especially when they first arrived, but Haylea appeared to have none.

CHAPTER FOURTEEN

DARK THOUGHTS

Having unpacked, Haylea came downstairs with me. She asked what she should do and I said whatever she liked.

'What do you normally do at this time?'

She shrugged, embarrassed. 'Nothing, really.'

'We'll have dinner at six when Paula is back from work,' I said. 'Would you like to read a book? I've got plenty you can borrow.'

'I find reading difficult,' she admitted. I wasn't surprised, as she'd missed so much school.

'I have some books that are easy to read. Would you like to try one?'

'No, thank you. Can I help you?'

'There's not a lot to do at present, love. Dinner is in the oven.'

'Can I watch television then?'

'Yes, of course.'

'I like watching television.' Which I also knew from the placement information form. It had been listed under hobbies and interests.

In the living room I showed Haylea how to work the remote control and she selected a children's channel aimed at six- to seven-year-olds.

'I love this programme,' she said, and her face lit up.

My heart went out to her.

I sat in one of the easy-chairs for a while with Darcy-May on my lap, watching Haylea. She was completely engrossed in the colourful animated cartoon. After a while I said, 'I'll be in the front room at the computer if you need me.'

She nodded without taking her eyes from the screen.

I took Darcy-May with me and sat her in the bouncing cradle while I checked emails with attachments. I find the attachments easier to read on the larger monitor of the computer rather than on my phone. I was still there when Paula arrived home at 5.45. I stopped what I was doing and asked her if she'd had a good day as she made a fuss of Darcy-May. 'Come and meet Haylea,' I said.

Paula carried Darcy-May into the living room where I introduced her to Haylea, who was still watching children's programmes.

'Hi, how are you?' Paula asked.

'OK,' Haylea replied shyly, then returned her attention to the television.

'Something smells good,' Paula said, sniffing the air.

'Vegetable and pasta bake. I'll put the garlic bread in now you're home.'

'I'll get changed.'

Paula liked to change from her office wear before dinner and she took Darcy-May upstairs with her. I left Haylea in the living room while I put the garlic bread in the oven. Ten minutes later dinner was ready and I called Paula and Haylea. Paula brought Darcy-May down and sat her in the bouncing cradle by the table so she could see us while we ate.

Paula is very easy-going and used to having others stay – I began fostering before she was born, so she's grown up with it. As we ate she did everything she could to put Haylea at ease and include her in the conversation – as did I – but Haylea remained awkward, self-conscious and shy. She was clearly uncomfortable meeting someone new and I guessed she was like that with everyone, probably one of the reasons she struggled to make friends at Waysbury.

As well as talking to Haylea, Paula and I kept Darcy-May amused during dinner. It would be another two months before I could start to wean her and introduce solid foods. As we ate she babbled, grinned and kicked her legs, but Haylea didn't look at her once and concentrated on eating. Paula was aware of Haylea's attitude to Darcy-May so just carried on as normal.

After dinner – Haylea ate well – Paula and Haylea cleared the table and loaded the dishwasher. Paula then said she was going to her room for a while. After she'd gone, Haylea began to talk again.

'Paula is nice,' she said.

'Yes. She is.'

'I like her.'

'Good.'

'Does she like me?'

'Yes.'

'Can I help you?'

'You have helped, thank you,' I replied. 'What do you like to do apart from watching television?'

She thought for a moment. 'Make cakes.'

'We can do that tomorrow. Anything else? Do you like listening to music?'

'Sometimes. Dylis put some on my phone, but I'd like to watch some more television now.'

'OK.'

I sat in the living room with her for a while and then left her watching television while I took Darcy-May upstairs for her bath and bed. Once I'd settled her in the cot, I returned to the living room where Haylea was still watching television. Paula joined us.

'Would you like a game of UNO?' she asked Haylea, referring to the card game. It was a lasting favourite of ours, as it is with many families, but I knew Paula was suggesting it now to try to engage Haylea. She didn't normally play cards in the evening after work.

'I don't know how to play it,' Haylea admitted.

'I'll show you,' Paula said, and fetched the box from the games cupboard in the kitchen-diner. Haylea recognized it. 'I saw some of them playing that at Waysbury,' she said.

'Yes, it's very popular,' I agreed.

Haylea silenced the television, Paula explained how to play the game and we began a tentative first round with me helping Haylea. The second round was easier for her and by the third she'd got the gist of it and had relaxed a little. True, there wasn't the laughing, exclamations and camaraderie there usually is when we play a game, but at least Haylea was joining in. Playing games and doing things together helps bond a family. We played for about half an hour and then Haylea said she was tired and would go to bed. It was only eight o'clock but I guessed she was exhausted from all the upheaval of the day.

Paula put away the cards and I asked Haylea if she wanted her bath now or in the morning.

'Tomorrow,' she said.

I went with her upstairs to make sure she had everything she needed and then left her to get ready. Once I heard her go into her bedroom, I went up to say goodnight. 'It's Cathy. Can I come in?' I asked, knocking on the bedroom door.

'Yes,' came her small voice.

She was in bed, peeping over the top of the duvet as a young child might. Her bedroom curtains were drawn, and it was still light outside.

'Is that how you like your curtains?' I asked. 'Pulled right to.'

'Yes.'

'That's fine then.'

On the first night I always ask the child or young person how they like to sleep: the curtains open or closed, the light on or off, the bedroom door open or shut. It's little familiar details like this that help them to settle in a strange room. It didn't matter that Haylea was fifteen. It would still take time before she felt at home. She wanted her light left on and the door closed.

'Can you switch off your phone for the night, please?' I said, seeing it on her bedside cabinet. 'So you have a good night's sleep.'

She did as I asked and snuggled down. 'Do you want a goodnight kiss?' I asked.

'I don't know,' she said. 'Is that what you normally do?'

I smiled. 'It depends. Some children like a hug and kiss goodnight, but others don't. I always ask.'

'Mum didn't kiss me when she was at home,' Haylea said, which I found incredibly sad.

'Shall I give you a little kiss on your forehead then?'

She nodded.

I kissed her forehead. 'Night, night, love, sleep tight.'

'Night,' she said. 'Thank you for having me. Will you say goodnight to Paula for me and tell her I like her?'

'Yes, of course, love.'

I came out, closing her bedroom door behind me, and went to Paula's room, where I told her what Haylea had said. She was as touched as I was but surprised at how little attention Haylea had given the baby. Although I'd previously told Paula what to expect, it wasn't until you saw the two of them together that it struck you.

'Perhaps she doesn't like the baby's father,' Paula suggested. 'Do you think she could have been raped?' she asked, grimacing.

'That occurred to me,' I said. 'It could explain why she has totally rejected Darcy-May. But at present Haylea's not saying.'

'Although she's fifteen, I feel very protective of her,' Paula said.

'Yes, I know exactly what you mean.'

Paula and I chatted for a while and then I returned downstairs and worked at my computer in the front room until it was time for bed.

I never sleep well when there is a new child in the house. I'm half awake, listening out, in case they wake, frightened, not knowing where they are and needing reassurance. It didn't matter that Haylea wasn't a young child. She was spending her first night in a strange house. But by morning I hadn't heard her, so I was hopeful she'd slept reasonably well.

However, when she came out of her room the following morning and I asked if she'd slept well, she replied, 'No. I never do.'

'Oh dear, I am sorry. Why not?'

'It's not your fault, Cathy. It's a nice room, but my head is full of bad thoughts. I can't switch them off at night.'

'What sort of bad thoughts?' I asked. We were on the landing. It was 8.30. I was dressed, but Haylea was in her pyjamas. Paula had left for work. 'Can you tell me what worries you at night?'

She shrugged. 'I get down. I can't shut the bad thoughts out. During the day it's better. If I watch television or do something, I don't have to think.'

'Those are distractions,' I said. 'When we have worries they are often worse at night. I think you are going to have to start talking to your therapist, don't you?'

'That's what Dylis said. Shall I have my bath now?' Haylea said, changing the subject.

'Yes. Shower or bath, it's up to you.'

'Bath. I like being in warm water.'

'It's comforting,' I agreed.

I checked Haylea had everything she needed and left her to have her bath, while I saw to Darcy-May. Haylea was in the bath for nearly an hour. I heard the hot water running as she topped up the water as it cooled. I checked on her a couple of times, knocking on the door, to make sure she was all right and hadn't fallen asleep. She clearly liked her bath, and while it was fine for her to have a leisurely soak in the morning now, it would be impractical when she began going to school again.

It was ten o'clock before Haylea appeared downstairs dressed. I made her the egg on toast she wanted for breakfast, and she poured herself a glass of juice. I joined her at the table with a coffee – I'd already had breakfast. Darcy-May was in her bouncing cradle, watching us. I was still thinking about Haylea lying awake at night.

'Have you tried listening to music at night if you can't sleep?' I suggested. 'Something mellow. It can help. I've got a CD of whale music that's supposed to be relaxing.'

Haylea stopped eating and looked at me. 'But I'm not a whale, Cathy,' she said.

I laughed. 'You could have fooled me with the amount of time you spent in the bath this morning!'

She laughed too. Despite all her problems, she had a sense of humour and I knew then we were going to get along just fine.

We baked and iced cupcakes that morning as Haylea wanted, then after lunch we went for a walk to our local park. It was a beautiful warm July day. I pushed Darcy-May in the stroller and Haylea walked beside us. Once there, Haylea played on the swings, roundabout and seesaw, then enjoyed feeding the ducks with the seed I'd brought from home. The following day we made a picnic lunch together and I drove to a local beauty spot and we picnicked by the river. The next day I took her to a famous street market in a neighbouring town. And so our days continued, easy, and as happy as Haylea could be with the burden she carried. If she wasn't fully occupied, I often saw her face cloud over as her thoughts returned to the demons that plagued her. Without doubt Haylea was a very troubled young person, but unless she began talking about it there was little I could do to help.

Our outings were curtailed a little by having Darcy-May so I couldn't, for example, take Haylea to the cinema as I would have liked to. But we did lots of other things, including visiting a local zoo. We went there at the weekend so Paula could join us. Haylea had never been to any of these places and was childlike in her enthusiasm. It was both touching and painful to see. So many of the children and young people I've fostered haven't had the opportunities my family and others have. It's a rewarding part of fostering that we can give the child these new experiences and it makes you appreciate your own upbringing.

Although Haylea still wasn't able to share her dark thoughts with me, I knew she was growing closer and bonding with me, faster than another young person might have. With no friends to socialize with and not being in school, she was with me all day and every day. Dylis and the cook from Waysbury texted her, but no one else had been in touch. The only time she was out alone was when she caught the bus to and from the counselling sessions. From the little she told me after-wards, she was talking to the therapist but not about anything that mattered. 'It's too difficult to go there,' she once said. I didn't press her. What happened between her and her therapist was private. Hopefully it would improve with time.

Haylea also became more relaxed around Paula, but when she met Adrian and Kirsty for the first time, and Lucy and her family, she recoiled into her shell again, wary and distrustful. Lucy, having been a foster child herself once, did all she could to put Haylea at ease, but she remained as wary of her as she was of all new people. Life experience must have taught her to be on guard with strangers. If I stopped to talk to someone in the street, I always introduced Haylea. She would say a shy hello and then move away and stand further up the pavement and wait for me to finish. I never talked for long and told Haylea that all the people I knew were nice.

Joy and Shari both made appointments to visit Haylea. They went through their usual business to make sure she was being well looked after and had everything she needed, and I updated them. Shari said she was arranging a review for Haylea the following week. When a child moves to a new placement a review is needed within four weeks. As Darcy-May's next review was due at the end of July, and they would both take place at my house, Shari decided to schedule them one after the other – Haylea's first and then Darcy-May's following on. Haylea had already had a review at Waysbury so knew what to expect. Shari said she hoped to have confirmation of Haylea's new school by then and Darcy-May's adoptive family, so it seemed everything was going as it should in the background. Both Joy and Shari remarked on how quickly Haylea had settled in, which I was pleased about. Joy also said I was doing a good job.

Although Haylea was bonding with me and Paula, she still managed to completely ignore Darcy-May. It was something I'd discussed with Joy and Shari and had cited this example: I had left Darcy-May in the living room with Haylea while I went into the kitchen to check on something in the oven. I was only gone a few moments but Darcy-May began to cry. Immediately Haylea appeared in the kitchen looking very anxious. 'It's crying,' she said, as if Darcy-May could harm her. I found her manner and the fact she'd called the baby 'it' quite unsettling. So did Joy and Shari; they were concerned.

My diary for the following week showed the reviews on Wednesday and Darcy-May's next vaccination on Thursday. The rest of the week was free, so I planned to fill it as I had been doing, by taking Haylea out each day and catching up on housework, writing and everything else in between. However, when we woke on Monday morning it was pouring with rain, absolutely tipping it down, so instead of going out as planned, Haylea and I baked. It was still raining heavily after lunch and Haylea watched some children's television while Darcy-May took a nap in her cot. I was limiting the amount of television Haylea was watching and was trying to get her interested in other activities, including reading some magazines, which she'd chosen while we'd been out shopping. I hadn't got her reading a book yet.

It suited me sometimes to let Haylea watch television so I could get on with something else. That Monday afternoon, while Darcy-May slept, I took the opportunity to work at my computer. The doors to the living room and front room were open and I could hear the television in the background. The baby monitor was beside me in the front room.

I was typing away, concentrating on the screen, when I became aware that it had gone quiet in the living room. I paused to listen. I couldn't hear the television any more, and neither could I hear Haylea moving around. She usually told me what she was doing or planning to do – 'I'm going to my room,' and so on.

'Haylea? Are you OK?' I called, my fingers hovering over the keyboard.

No reply.

'Haylea?'

Nothing. Not a sound.

Concerned and puzzled, I stood and went down the hall. The door to the living room was still open and I went in. Haylea was on the sofa where I'd left her, faced away, the remote control in her hand, but the television was switched off.

'Haylea, are you OK?'

It was only when she turned to face me that I saw the tears running silently down her cheeks.

'Oh, love, whatever is the matter?'

CHAPTER FIFTEEN

SICKENING DISCLOSURES

Haylea didn't reply. I sat beside her on the sofa and took her hand in mine.

'What is it, love? What's upset you?' I didn't put my arm around her as I might have with a different child as she was still uncomfortable with hugs if I initiated them. 'Tell me, love. What's upset you?'

She sniffed, and I passed her the box of tissues I kept on the coffee table.

'There was a programme on just now about a children's party,' she said, dabbing her eyes.

'Yes?' I prompted. 'Why has that upset you?'

'You know that address I gave you when I was at Waysbury?'

'Yes. The police went but there weren't any children living there.'

'I know, Shari told me. It was the right address, but the children aren't there all the time. They don't live there. They only go when there is a party. But they're not nice parties, not like you see on the television.'

'Can you explain, love?' I asked, suddenly feeling cold.

'Oh, Cathy, I can't tell you!' she cried. 'You'll think me a really bad person, wicked.'

'No, I won't. If something is worrying you, which clearly it is, you need to share it.'

Haylea pulled and twisted the tissue she was holding, making it tear, then took a deep breath. 'The man who lives at that address has parties. Children are taken there and the men do bad things to them.' Her tears had stopped and her voice was flat, emotionless and detached. 'I'm telling you because I want you to help them, but I can't tell anyone else because they'll kill me. The men made us do things to them and they did things to us. I got hurt, so did the children. I don't care about me, but those other kids, they were younger than me.'

I stared at her, my thoughts racing and my heart thumping loudly. Did I believe her? Yes, her manner and the way she'd said it. I'd known all along she had secrets, but nothing had prepared me for this. I felt physically sick, but I knew I had to stay calm for Haylea's sake. It wouldn't help her if I went to pieces.

'Will you tell someone so the children can be saved?' she said. 'Don't say it was me or they will hurt me more.' I felt her hand trembling in mine.

'They won't hurt you,' I said, struggling to keep my voice even. 'You've been very brave to tell me. I will phone your social worker and tell her, but she and the police will need to hear it from you too. How often did this happen?' I asked, feeling I should get a bit more information before I spoke to Shari.

'Every few weeks,' Haylea said. 'I hated going there but he forced me to.'

'Who?'

'Him, my father,' she said, struggling to use the word. 'I know I'm a dirty little cow. You'll hate me now you know. He said I enjoyed it, but I didn't.' Fresh tears formed and she laid her head on my shoulder.

'Oh, love, of course I don't hate you. You were abused, a victim of evil men. Your father and the others involved need to be stopped and punished.'

'I don't care about me, but those little kids,' she said again. 'That's why I'm telling you.'

'I understand. You've done well.'

'They called them parties, but they weren't real parties, were they?'

'No.'

'I had to go there on my birthday last year and the year before. He – my father – said I'd be given presents and play games, but I wasn't given any presents, and the games I had to play were horrible. It was even worse because it was my birthday. They said it was a special treat, but I hated it. That's why I don't like birthdays.'

Haylea had said before that bad things happened on her birthday without saying what, but I'd heard enough. Clearly if what she was saying was true, as I believed it to be, then she and others had been sexually abused by paedophiles. While I didn't need to hear any more, now she'd finally begun talking about it the words poured out.

'They gave us alcohol,' she said in the same flat, dispassionate voice. 'Even those little kids. They took us into the bedrooms and then they would swap. The little kids used to cry, but I learnt not to, it just made it worse. He would stuff things in my mouth and tape it shut while he did things to me.'

'Who?'

'Him, my father. The other men used to watch, then take turns. Sometimes they had another child in the room, and they would do things to us at the same time. He said I was old enough and to shut up making a fuss, but it still hurt. I think they have damaged me, Cathy. Sometimes when I go to the toilet it hurts so much.'

I'd heard children disclose sexual abuse before – sadly, most foster cares have – but it had been a long time since I'd heard anything this bad. I was shocked, upset and disgusted.

'Sometimes at night I can hear those children crying like they did in that house,' Haylea said. 'He – my father – told me they liked the little kids as they were tighter.'

I struggled to hide my revulsion and distress.

'They are evil,' I said. 'Do you know who the children are? Their names or where they live?'

'No, but I heard one of them call the man who owned the house "Uncle". She was crying and begging him to stop, she said, "Please, Uncle, don't, I promise to be good …" I wanted to tell someone, Cathy, really I did, but I knew they would kill me if I did. I'm scared. Do you hate me?'

'No, of course I don't hate you. Far from it. You and those other children have been badly abused.'

'Have I been abused, Cathy?' she asked naively.

'Yes. You have.' It seemed the abuse had become so much a part of Haylea's life that she hadn't recognized it for what it was.

'My father said he did those things because he loved me.'

'That's not a father's love, it's abuse,' I said vehemently. 'Now I need to phone Shari.'

'You will stay with me, won't you?' she asked, gripping my arm.

'Yes, love.'

I reached out and picked up my mobile phone from the coffee table and with my hand trembling I called Shari's number. It went through to her voicemail, so I left a message. 'It's Cathy Glass. Haylea has just disclosed shocking sexual abuse. I'll call your office number.'

I phoned her office and a colleague answered. 'It's Cathy, Haylea Walsh's carer. I need to speak to Shari urgently.'

'She's not in the office,' he said. 'I think she's on a home visit.'

'How long is she likely to be? I've left a message on her voicemail. It is urgent,' I emphasized.

'Shall I contact her and ask her to call you?'

'Yes, please, as soon as possible.'

As the call ended I heard Darcy-May crying loudly from her cot upstairs. Usually I got to her as soon as she woke, but the baby monitor was in the front room and I'd been concentrating on Haylea.

'I need to see to Darcy-May,' I said to Haylea. 'Will you be all right for a moment?'

She nodded. My heart went out to her. She looked utterly wretched but was being so brave. I took my phone with me in case Shari returned my call straight away and hurried upstairs and into my bedroom. Because I hadn't answered Darcy-May's calls immediately she had worked herself into quite a lather and was red in the face.

'Sshh, it's OK,' I soothed, picking her up. Instantly her crying stopped. 'That's better.'

Her nappy was full, so I changed it. Once she was clean, I held her close and began downstairs. With another stab of horror, I now understood why Haylea had rejected Darcy-May. Her baby most probably wasn't the result of a relationship or even a one-night stand, but the result of being repeatedly raped by a paedophile gang, one of whom was likely to be her father. It was truly shocking. But I then had another distressing thought. Haylea's father had been one of her abusers, so there was a chance that Darcy-May was the result of incest and she and Haylea had the same biological father. Struggling to maintain my composure, I held Darcy-May closer still and continued downstairs and into the living room.

'Are you all right, love?' I asked, my breath short. 'I'm just going to get a bottle for Darcy-May.' Haylea was still sitting on the sofa as I'd left her, staring into space.

'Yes,' she replied.

'Do you want a drink?' I asked her.

'No, thank you.'

I thought she was taking all this remarkably well, but then she'd been living with the abuse for – how long? She'd mentioned two birthdays so at least two years, probably longer. The poor child.

In the kitchen I warmed a bottle of formula and then returned to the living room and sat beside Haylea.

'You're doing very well,' I said to her as I began to feed Darcy-May.

'I don't feel like I am.'

My mobile rang. It was Shari. I answered, lodging the phone between my neck and shoulder so I could talk and still feed Darcy-May.

'What's happened?' Shari asked. 'I got your message.' Usually composed, I could hear the anxiety in her voice.

'Haylea has disclosed appalling sexual abuse at the hands of what sounds like a paedophile ring, which included her father.'

'Oh no. Is she all right?'

'She's with me now. She's being very brave. She says other children were involved and could still be being hurt now. The abuse happened at the address Haylea gave us, but the children don't live there. They are taken there to be abused.'

'Shit. The police must have missed that,' Shari said. 'Can I speak to Haylea?'

'Shari wants to talk to you,' I said, and passed her my phone.

I couldn't hear what Shari said, but Haylea answered her questions in a small, deadpan voice. 'Yes ... No ... I don't know ... I think so.'

I continued to feed Darcy-May.

After a few minutes Haylea said a quiet goodbye and, ending the call, returned the phone to the coffee table. 'Shari said to tell you she will come here with a police officer.'

'Do you know when?'

'She said later today.'

'OK, love.'

'I'm scared,' Haylea said.

'I know, but you're safe now. Just tell Shari and the police what you have told me.'

'There's other stuff,' Haylea said. 'But I can't tell you.'

'I understand. But it's important you tell Shari and the officer so those evil men can be caught and prosecuted.'

She nodded and then sat quietly staring into space as though she were far away.

I didn't need to hear any more to know that Haylea had suffered shocking abuse. I was aware of some of the atrocities that paedophiles committed from some foster-carer training I'd attended. The content had haunted me for months. I can still remember one harrowing scene from a video we'd been shown where a paedophile had been interviewed by the police and tried to defend his actions. It had upset and sickened me but made me more aware. It had also prepared me for when a child I was fostering disclosed sexual abuse, so I didn't go to pieces. There are paedophiles in all societies and being aware helps us protect our vulnerable children.

That afternoon was one of the longest of my life as the minutes slowly ticked by and we waited for Shari and the police to arrive.

'Can I have the television on?' Haylea asked after a while.

'Yes, of course, love.'

She switched it on and I stayed with her in the living room with Darcy-May on my lap while she watched a children's programme.

Did Darcy-May look like Haylea's abuser? I wondered, as we sat there. It would have been insensitive of me to ask. I could see some likeness between Darcy-May and Haylea, especially around the eyes. But what did Haylea see? Her father or another abuser? She'd barely looked at Darcy-May since that first meeting at the Family Centre. She'd asked to see her and had wanted to take a photograph but had then changed her mind. Had she seen her abuser mirrored in her baby's face? Is that why she had totally rejected her and couldn't even bare to look at her? If so, it was surprising she'd wanted to live with me, but then again, she'd managed to block out Darcy-May, probably as she'd had to block out years of abuse in order to survive. Would Haylea ever be able to see Darcy-May for the adorable baby she was without thinking of her abuser? I had no idea.

I touched Haylea's arm and she didn't recoil. 'Are you OK? You're doing very well.'

'Am I, Cathy?' she asked quietly, glancing at me.

'Yes, love. You're being very brave.'

'I don't feel brave,' she said. 'I'm a mess.'

She returned her attention to the television and I watched it too for a few minutes. I could see how the brightly coloured, fast-moving children's programmes could distract her from the reality of life. They drew you in.

Darcy-May began to gurgle at Haylea, trying to attract her attention, but she remained oblivious to her. So fragile, innocent and unaware of the horror of her conception – would Darcy-May ever learn of her past? I didn't know, but certainly she must never feel ashamed. I loved Darcy-May and felt very protective of her, and Haylea. I would do all I could to help them both.

At 5.30, when we'd heard nothing further from Shari, I suggested to Haylea we made something for dinner. She usually liked to cook so I thought it might help occupy her.

'I'm not hungry,' she said.

'Neither am I, but we need to eat, and Paula will be home in half an hour.'

'Will you tell Paula what I've told you?' Haylea asked.

'Only that you have disclosed abuse. Is that all right? Otherwise she will wonder why the police are here.'

'Yes, that's OK.'

I persuaded Haylea to come with me into the kitchen where I sat Darcy-May in her bouncing cradle. I began opening and closing cupboard doors, then the fridge and freezer, looking for some inspiration as to what we could have for dinner. My mind just wasn't on it.

'Come on, Haylea,' I said. 'Tell me what we can make. What did Cook used to make for your dinner?'

'Lot of things,' Haylea replied.

'Like what? What was your favourite meal?'

At that moment the front doorbell rang and Haylea froze.

'It's all right, just take a deep breath. I'll answer it.'

I picked up Darcy-May and, leaving Haylea in the kitchen, I went to the front door. Shari and two police officers greeted me with serious, sombre expressions. I showed them into the living room and then fetched Haylea.

'I recognize you,' the female officer said to Haylea.

'Are you the police officer who came to my house?' she asked.

'Yes.'

'I hoped you would help me, but you didn't.'

'I'm so sorry,' the officer replied, and she looked it.

CHAPTER SIXTEEN

A MONSTER FOR A FATHER

As we sat in the living room and talked, I learnt that the police officer, DC Jo Spar, had visited Haylea's father two years ago. Haylea had been in the living room when Jo had first arrived. Jo was a uniformed officer then – not CID – and had gone there to speak to Haylea's father about a stolen car. She remembered she'd asked Haylea why she wasn't in school and her father had said she was ill, then told her to go to her room to rest. That was the only contact Jo had had with Haylea, but Haylea remembered being in her bedroom, trying to summon the courage to go downstairs and tell Jo what was happening to her, but she was too scared. She hoped the officer would realize and rescue her, but of course Jo had no reason to suspect she was being abused.

'Couldn't you have told a teacher, a friend or an adult you trusted?' Jo now asked Haylea.

'I didn't have any friends and didn't go to school much,' Haylea replied. Often it's a teacher at school who first raises concern if they suspect a child is being abused or neglected at home. 'I didn't know any adults I could trust,' Haylea added.

Jo nodded sombrely. While that police visit two years

ago could be said to be a missed opportunity, it wasn't Jo's fault, although she apologized again. 'I am sorry,' she said.

She then asked Haylea about the 'parties' and the abuse she was claiming she'd suffered, and Haylea told her what she'd told me. Jo's colleague made some notes. Jo asked Haylea questions about the house where the parties were held, dates and times, and the adults and other children present. Haylea answered as best she could and revealed more details of the shocking abuse, which were too graphic to describe here. Darcy-May had fallen asleep in my lap by now and I concentrated on her as Haylea talked about the many times her father had abused her at home and also taken her to other houses to be abused. Her voice was flat and dispassionate. It was truly the stuff of nightmares and I wondered how she had survived at all. It seemed it had been going on for seven years, since she was about eight years old, all set up and orchestrated by her father. It was the worst case of abuse I'd ever come across. And as I sat there, I thought the only way to describe Haylea's father was as a monster.

Jo and her colleague managed to keep their expressions neutral and maintain a professional detachment as Haylea described what had been done to her and the other children, but Shari was visibly upset and left the room at one point to get a glass of water.

At six o'clock I heard the front door open as Paula returned home from work. I excused myself and went into the hall. 'The police are interviewing Haylea,' I said quietly. 'I'm not sure how long we'll be.'

'Shall I take Darcy-May?' Paula offered. She was still asleep in my arms.

'Thanks, love, she can go in her cot for now.' I passed her to Paula and returned to the living room and to more details of Haylea's horrific suffering at the hands of her father and other men.

Jo asked Haylea about the other children. But apart from one of them calling the man who owned the house "Uncle", Haylea said she didn't know any more and couldn't give a description. 'When they were in the room they put a bag over my head so I couldn't see them,' Haylea said, and my stomach lurched.

'They could have been his niece and nephew,' Jo said. 'Or possibly it was a term the children had to use. Did you have to call those men "Uncle"?' she asked Haylea.

'No,' she replied. 'I was told not to say anything and to do what they wanted. If I didn't, it was worse for me and I was punished.' She then described the punishments, which were just another way of abusing her. It was horrendous, depraved, and I struggled to believe any human being could do that to another, let alone to a child.

It was nearly 7 p.m. when the police finally wound up and prepared to leave.

'What happens now?' Haylea asked.

'We will speak to your father and also the man at the address you gave us,' Jo said. 'Then take it from there.'

'Will they be arrested?' Haylea asked.

'It's likely. We will need you to come into the police station to make a statement.'

'I won't have to see them, will I?' Haylea asked.

'No.'

Shari stayed with Haylea in the living room while I saw the police officers out. I could hear Paula upstairs tending to Darcy-May, who was awake now. I returned to the living room where Shari was trying to reassure Haylea that her father couldn't do her any more harm.

'What about the others?' she asked.

'If you ever see any of them while you are out, tell Cathy or call the police,' Shari said.

'I'll take you to counselling in the car,' I said. It was the only time Haylea went out alone.

'I haven't got a session this week, she's on holiday,' Haylea said.

'All right,' Shari said. 'You'll need to have a medical. I'll arrange it.'

'I don't want another one!' Haylea cried. 'The infection has gone.'

'But you said earlier you were in pain when you went to the toilet,' I reminded her.

'I am sometimes.'

'I think you should get it checked,' I said.

'I don't want to. The doctor at the hospital said there was something wrong when I had the baby, but I didn't understand.'

'Shall I phone the hospital and talk to the doctor?' Shari suggested. Haylea nodded and Shari made a note. 'But if your condition gets any worse, you need to see a doctor.'

'OK,' Haylea agreed.

'Do you have any questions?' Shari asked her, and Haylea shook her head. 'Do you have everything you need here?'

'Yes,' she replied.

'I'll phone as soon as I have any news,' Shari said, and packed away her notepad and pen.

I saw Shari out. She looked pale and drawn as she left, which was hardly surprising considering the disclosures Haylea had just made. As I closed the front door Paula came downstairs with Darcy-May in her arms and a half-empty bottle of formula. 'I gave her some feed. I hope that was right.'

'Yes, thanks, love.' I was grateful – my routine was all out.

'Are you OK?' Paula asked me. I guess I was looking rough as well.

'That poor child,' I said quietly, referring to Haylea. 'The things she's been through.'

Paula didn't need to know the gruesome details of Haylea's suffering and she didn't ask.

'Shall I make us some dinner?' she offered.

'We'll have something quick.'

Haylea came out of the living room. 'I'm going to my bedroom,' she said.

'OK, love. I'll tell you when dinner is ready.'

She said hi to Paula and went slowly upstairs. Paula and I went into the kitchen where we sat Darcy-May in her bouncing cradle. I took some curry I'd previously made from the freezer and reheated it as Paula boiled some fresh rice. Once it was ready, I went upstairs to fetch Haylea. Her bedroom door was slightly open, so I knocked and went in. She was sitting on her bed concentrating on her phone.

'Dylis texted me,' she said.

'Oh yes?'

'She said to make sure I tell the police everything. But how did she know they were coming?'

'You didn't tell her?' I checked.

'No.'

'I guess the police or Shari must have spoken to someone at Waysbury, as it's the last place you lived before coming to me. They will be gathering information. Did you tell Dylis or anyone there about the abuse?'

'No. I only told you.'

'All right. Don't worry. I am sure Dylis knows it's confidential.'

I thought it was a bit insensitive and unprofessional, though, for Dylis to have sent this text, making Haylea aware that she knew of the abuse. Of course, how much Dylis had been told and in what context I didn't know. Haylea seemed reassured and she came with me downstairs for dinner.

As usual the three of us ate at the table in the kitchen-diner while Darcy-May watched from her bouncing cradle. I didn't have much appetite and I was preoccupied and kept glancing at Haylea to check she was coping. We didn't have to make conversation as Darcy-May, refreshed from her sleep, was very vocal and babbled continuously. Paula and I smiled and replied, but Haylea, as usual, managed to ignore her. Haylea's face was expressionless, as it often was. But I now knew it was masking unimaginable pain from years of abuse, which would have to find its way out before she could start to heal. I thought it was a pity her counselling session for this week had been cancelled. She needed more, not less.

After dinner I took Darcy-May up for her bath, later than usual because of the police visit. Haylea watched television in the living room. When I came down from settling Darcy-May in her cot Haylea said she was going to have an early night. I asked her how she was and she said, 'OK,' in a blank, emotionless tone. I was struggling to believe she was functioning at all with all she'd been through.

Once Haylea was in bed, I checked on her. 'Are you all right?' I asked.

'Yes,' she replied. 'But Dylis has sent me some more messages. She is asking what I told the police.'

'You don't have to tell her,' I said. 'It was different when you lived at Waysbury. She was your key worker then.'

'I've told her I don't want to talk about it,' Haylea said. 'Will she think I'm rude?'

'No, love. She doesn't need to know. If she keeps texting and it becomes a problem, tell me and I will speak to Fran. But I want you to switch off your phone soon anyway so you can get some sleep.'

Haylea switched it off there and then. 'Call me if you need me in the night,' I said, and, saying goodnight, I came out, closing her bedroom door. I doubted she'd sleep much, and neither would I with everything so fresh. Downstairs Paula and I had a cup of tea together in the living room while watching the news and then we both went to bed.

Of course I couldn't sleep, and Darcy-May, having had her routine disrupted, woke three times during the night. I also heard Haylea get up to use the toilet, so I went round the landing and asked her if she was all right.

'Yes, thank you,' she said. 'You're always so kind to me.' She broke my heart.

Finally it was morning and Darcy-May woke for a feed at 6.30. Once I'd fed and changed her, I settled her in her cot, then showered and dressed. There was no telling what was going to happen today, so I wanted to be up and ready. As I went downstairs I could hear Paula getting up. I fed Sammy, put the kettle on and some bread in the toaster. Paula and I usually had toast and a hot drink for breakfast on a week day. Darcy-May was asleep again in her cot and I assumed Haylea was still asleep. However, a few minutes later, as the toaster popped, I heard movement coming from her room. It's directly above the kitchen. Her bedroom door opened and she came downstairs.

'You're up early, love,' I began as she came into the kitchen. I stopped as her face crumpled. 'What is it, love?' I asked, going to her.

'I'm so upset. I've just turned on my phone and Dylis is being horrible to me.'

'What? Let me see.'

She passed me her phone and I looked at the messages. Dylis had been texting all night, although she hadn't received any replies, as Haylea's phone had been switched off. I saw the one from last night when she'd asked Haylea what she'd told the police, and Haylea had replied that she didn't want to talk about it. Then she'd switched off her phone and Dylis had texted:

Why don't you want to talk to me about it?

Receiving no reply, Dylis had continued:

Why? Tell me.

Why aren't you answering?

If you don't tell me, I'll think you made it up.

You're just trying to get attention.

We all have problems. Yours are no worse than anyone else's.

Why aren't you texting back?

The last message read: *You're a liar.*

I looked up, shocked. 'I can't believe she's done this,' I said to Haylea. 'It's completely out of order and untrue.' I wondered if Dylis had been drunk or under the influence of drugs. Even so, there was no excuse. Not only was it unprofessional and inaccurate, it suggested Dylis had mental-health issues of her own – the last person to be looking after vulnerable young people!

'I'll telephone Fran,' I said to Haylea. 'Don't upset yourself. This says more about Dylis than you. Ignore it and don't text back.'

'I didn't make it up,' Haylea said.

'I know you didn't. So do the police and Shari. How was Dylis with you when you lived at Waysbury?' I asked.

'OK, I guess,' Haylea said, with a shrug. 'When I first arrived she used to ask me a lot of questions about my past and why I was there, but when I didn't tell her she got fed up and talked to others.'

It was very worrying. 'I'll speak to Fran.'

'Shall I delete the messages?' Haylea asked as I handed back her phone.

'No, leave them for now in case someone wants to see them.'

Haylea poured herself a glass of water and returned upstairs to her room. I was still reeling from the messages. Whatever had Dylis been thinking? It was only 7.30 a.m. but I telephoned Waysbury. Their answerphone cut in, so I left a message. 'It's Cathy Glass. Could Fran call me, please, as soon as possible? It's important.'

I would try again at 8 a.m. and then every half an hour until I spoke to Fran or someone there in authority. My main concern now was for the other young people at Waysbury who Dylis was responsible for. Haylea had been upset, but she was safely away from Dylis and knew that her messages had been wrong and entirely inappropriate. I'd speak to her again later, but what of the other young people at Waysbury? Was Dylis with them now? Had she been on night duty when she'd sent her messages?

What a start to the day! I thought. As if we didn't already have enough to deal with.

Paula came downstairs for breakfast and I didn't worry her with this latest development. I sat at the table with her, sipping my coffee while she had toast and tea, then she went upstairs to finish getting ready for work. I phoned Waysbury again at eight o'clock and the answerphone cut in, so I left another message. Five minutes later my mobile rang and it was Fran.

'Good morning, Cathy. I've just picked up your messages. It sounds urgent.'

'Yes, it is. Was Dylis on night duty last night?'

'Yes, why?'

I told her about all the text messages she'd sent Haylea.

There was silence and then Fran said sombrely, 'I'll speak to her now. No, on second thoughts, let me speak to Haylea first.'

'Just a minute. She's upstairs.'

I took my phone up to Haylea's room. 'Fran wants to talk to you,' I said, knocking on her door and going in. 'It's about Dylis,' I added, passing her the phone.

I waited on the landing in case I was needed as Haylea answered Fran's questions and then read out all the messages from last night. Paula called goodbye from the hall as she left.

'Bye, love. Have a good day,' I said, going to the top of the stairs so I could see her.

'And you,' she replied, and blew me a kiss.

Darcy-May was now awake so I went to my bedroom. As I was changing her nappy Haylea appeared, having finished talking to Fran.

'Fran said to tell you she is going to phone you once she's spoken to Dylis.'

'Thanks, love. Are you all right?'

'Fran believes me.'

'Of course she does. So do I. It was very wrong of Dylis to send you those messages. Very wrong indeed.'

'Why do you think she did it?'

'I don't know. But if she contacts you again, tell me straight away.'

'I will. Thank you for looking after me,' Haylea said again.

'You're welcome, love.' I smiled.

However, it wasn't Haylea who Dylis contacted. It was me, although I didn't know who it was to begin with.

CHAPTER SEVENTEEN

I PRETEND

I was in the living room with Darcy-May when a text arrived on my phone, from a number I didn't recognize.

You have ruined my life! I hate you. You fucking cow.

I was stunned and upset that anyone could think so badly of me. I sat for a moment wondering who it could be and not knowing what to do for the best. After a while, and with trembling hands, I texted back: *Who is this?*

The reply was instant. I could feel her rage. *Dylis. I've lost my fucking job because of you. I hope you die. You bitch.*

I didn't reply but I telephoned Waysbury. I was concerned that Dylis could be with young people now. Fran answered and I told her of Dylis's texts to me.

'Oh dear. I spoke to Dylis about the messages she sent to Haylea,' Fran said. 'She left in a state and I am trying to contact her parents. She hasn't lost her job, but I have put her on sick leave and told her to see her doctor. She's clearly not well.'

'All right. I won't keep you then.'

The matter had been dealt with.

I briefly wondered how Dylis had got my number. I supposed that as a key worker she had access to the children's files, or possibly Haylea had given it to her. It didn't matter, and I hoped that Dylis would do as Fran asked and see her doctor.

Once Haylea was dressed, she came downstairs and I made her breakfast, then sat with her while she ate it. I didn't tell her of Dylis's text messages to me. There was no need.

'What shall we do today?' she asked as she ate.

'What would you like to do? We won't go too far away in case we're needed by Shari or the police.'

'Let's go to the park and feed the ducks,' she suggested. 'Perhaps Lucy can come and we'll have a family outing.'

I smiled. 'Good idea.'

'We could take a picnic.'

'Yes.'

Haylea seemed much brighter now she had been able to tell us of her abuse, as though a huge weight had been lifted from her shoulders. As she finished her breakfast I telephoned Lucy and asked her if she'd like to come to the park with us for a picnic. She said she'd be with us in about an hour. 'Also, Mum, I was going to phone you. Emma's first birthday. We're doing a little party here on Saturday. Just family.'

'Fantastic. Tell me what I can do to help.'

'Nothing. You just come. See you soon.'

Haylea wanted to make the picnic so I helped her gather together the items we needed from the cupboards and fridge – cheese, ham, rolls, crisps, salad and so forth, and then left her to make it. I prepared bottles of formula to take with us and then checked I had everything I needed in the baby bag. I also found the bag containing the ground sheet for us to sit on.

Lucy arrived at 11.30 and we set off up the road. 'We're on a family outing,' Haylea said more than once – something she'd had very little experience of as a child.

It was another lovely warm summer day, just right for a picnic, and I was glad Haylea had suggested it. She asked Lucy if she could push Emma in the stroller and then chatted to Emma as we walked. Once in the park, she wanted to push her in the baby swing and then sit with her on the roundabout.

'Haylea seems a bit better,' Lucy said quietly to me.

'Yes. She's disclosed a lot of abuse. The poor girl has been through so much. The police are involved.'

'Oh no,' Lucy said. She didn't say any more and neither did I. We didn't have to.

Lucy made a point of talking to Haylea as she had before – about television programmes, boy bands and so on – although in truth they didn't have that much in common. This time Haylea was far more responsive and replied. She wasn't easy in company, although she was improving. However, it didn't escape my notice that she was taking an interest in Emma in a way she never did with Darcy-May. Part of that could have been that a one-year-old was more responsive and interesting than a four-month-old baby, but of course that wasn't the real reason. When Haylea looked at Emma all she saw was a cute toddler – unconnected to her past suffering.

When it was lunchtime I spread the ground sheet in the shade of a tree, and Haylea proudly arranged the boxes of food she'd prepared in the centre. She then handed out the plastic plates, napkins and cartons of juice. Lucy spoon-fed Emma the mashed-up food she'd brought with her and for dessert gave her sliced fruit, which Emma made a good attempt at feeding to herself. As we ate Lucy told me what she was planning for Emma's first birthday party.

'Two o'clock at our place. I'll do a buffet,' she said. 'I've texted Adrian and Kirsty, and Paula. Darren's family will be there too.'

'Can I come?' Haylea asked.

'Yes, of course,' Lucy said. 'I assumed you would if you're free.'

'I'm always free,' Haylea said with an edge of sadness. 'I don't have friends to go out with.'

'You will,' I said. 'Once you start school, you'll make friends. You can invite them home for tea and sleep-overs if you wish.'

Her face lit up. 'I will,' she said.

Moments like this confirmed why I fostered. I was making a difference and helping Haylea to a better future. However, I knew we had a long way to go. Haylea had been able to disclose horrendous abuse, but that wouldn't be enough to exorcize her past. It would take years, and therapy, and hopefully the conviction of those responsible. But at least it was a start.

We stayed in the park until nearly three o'clock and then strolled home. Lucy came in for a while and left around four o'clock. I hadn't heard anything from the social services or the police, and Haylea's and Darcy-May's reviews were the following day. I was wondering if they were still going ahead so I emailed Shari and she replied they were. Then Joy phoned, apologized for not being in contact as she'd been sorting out 'an emergency placement' and asked if Haylea had been to the police station yet to make her statement. I said she hadn't.

That night Haylea had a nightmare. I was woken just after 2 a.m. by a chilling scream. I was out of bed in a heartbeat and going round the landing to her room. Her door opened and she came out.

'He's in there!' she cried, grabbing my arm.

She was petrified, hot and hyperventilating.

'There's no one there,' I said. I raised the light in her bedroom. 'Look. Your room is empty. You're safe.'

She was still clutching my arm and looked as though she'd seen a ghost. 'You had a nightmare, a bad dream.'

She was disorientated and kept agitatedly licking her lips. 'Come and see, there is no one in your room.'

She allowed me to draw her in; on guard and watchful, she ran her gaze over the room. 'You're safe,' I said again. 'The room is empty.'

'Who else is in this house?' she asked.

'Just me and Paula.'

'There are no men here?'

'No, love.'

'And my father doesn't know where I am.'

'No.'

'He's not here?'

'No. You're safe. You had a bad dream.'

Finally, she began to relax and let go of my arm.

'It seemed so real. I thought he was here.'

'I know, love.'

'I was sure he was here and hurting me.' She stopped, the memory too painful to verbalize.

'I understand. You're OK,' I said.

174

Eventually she felt able to go back to bed. I sat with her for a while and then said, 'Try to go to sleep now. I'll be in my room if you need me.'

'Thank you. Leave the light up high. Are all the doors locked?'

'Yes. You're safe.'

I waited for a few moments longer and then returned to my bedroom, although I didn't immediately fall asleep. I listened to the steady rhythm of Darcy-May's light breathing and thought of Haylea's night terror. It would happen again for sure, if not tonight then another night. Now she was starting to talk about the abuse, which her mind had suppressed for so long in order for her to survive, it would keep resurfacing until it was dealt with. Dreaming is one of the ways the brain cleanses itself.

Thankfully Paula and Darcy-May hadn't been woken by Haylea's scream. An hour later I checked on Haylea and she was asleep. However, the following morning when she woke the nightmare was still fresh in her mind.

'It was so real,' she said, coming to find me. 'I thought he was there in my room and it was all happening again. I could feel him on me, doing things just like he used to.'

'Who?'

'Him – my father. I could smell him and hear him panting.' She shuddered. 'It was dreadful.'

'I know, love, but you're safe here. That can't happen any more.'

'You're sure he doesn't know I'm living here?'

'Positive. Ask Shari when we see her this afternoon.'

There was no reason for her father to have my contact details and as far as I knew he didn't, but the hospital had accidently divulged my address to Haylea. I didn't point this out to her and I thought her father would have shown up by now causing trouble if he was going to. Hopefully he would be in police custody before long.

Haylea's review was set for two o'clock that afternoon and Darcy-May's at three. Reviews are usually an hour long. We needed some more milk, so that morning I suggested we walk to the local shop. Haylea was quieter than she had been yesterday during our visit to the park.

'Are you all right, love?' I asked her.

She shrugged. 'I keep thinking about everything that happened to me. I don't want to, but the thoughts keep coming into my head. Things I'd forgotten. I can't shut them out.'

'It's because you feel safe now that your mind is allowing you to remember. It will improve with time, but you need to tell your therapist when you see her. She might have some strategies for managing these unwanted thoughts.'

'I hope so.'

From my experience of looking after other children who'd disclosed abuse, I knew it would probably be months, if not years, before these intrusive thoughts stopped or at least improved. There was only so much help I could give Haylea and it needed a qualified therapist, and again I thought it was a pity the session this week had been cancelled.

We bought the milk and a few other food items we fancied and then returned home for lunch. After we'd eaten I put Darcy-May in her cot upstairs for an afternoon nap. I placed the receiver for the baby monitor in the living room where we would be gathering for the review.

Reviews can be quite formal, although less so if the child is present. They usually begin in a quiet, orderly manner when everyone who is attending is seated and the IRO (Independent Reviewing Officer) asks us to introduce ourselves. Not so with Haylea's review.

Shari arrived fifteen minutes early as she wanted to update Haylea before the review. She walked briskly into the living room, where she perched on the sofa next to Haylea and began to tell us that yesterday the police went to the address Haylea had given them. 'They searched the house and arrested the man living there,' she said. I didn't hear any more as the front doorbell rang.

I left Shari and Haylea and answered the door. It was Joy, who always liked to arrive a few minutes early for a review. I showed her through to the living room where Shari paused from talking to Haylea to ask Joy if the children had been placed.

'Yes. I've emailed you the details,' she replied.

'Thank you,' Shari said, and returned her attention to Haylea. Joy sat on a chair close by.

'Where's Darcy-May?' she asked me.

'Upstairs having a nap.'

I didn't know who the children were Shari had referred to, but if it was relevant to Haylea or Darcy-May it should be included in her report to the review.

The doorbell rang again and I left the room. It was Jasmine Patel, the Education Welfare Officer for the county. I knew her from when she'd been involved with other children I'd fostered. Her role was to make sure young people in the area were being educated, especially those like Haylea whose schooling had been disrupted.

'How are you?' I asked her as she came in.

'Good. Sorry I haven't been in touch before about Haylea. I've just got back from holiday.'

'I hope you had a good time,' I said as I showed her into the living room. Shari and Joy both knew her and she'd met Haylea at Waysbury, so they all said hello to each other and I offered everyone a drink.

'A coffee would be lovely, thank you,' Shari said.

'Just water, please,' Jasmine said.

Joy and Haylea didn't want anything.

I went into the kitchen to make the drinks as Sammy disappeared through the cat flap. He usually stayed if there were just a couple of visitors, but any more and he left to find a quieter place outside. I didn't know who else had been invited to the review, only that no one from Haylea's family had been. Haylea and I had received the invitations to the review the week before and had completed our review forms online. The hum of conversation drifted in.

I made the drinks and took them into the living room. Shari was still talking to Haylea and Joy, and Jasmine was listening intently. I guessed there'd been a number of developments since the police had visited us on Monday, and from the snatches I'd heard at least one arrest had been made. Shari would update us all at the review.

It was now exactly 2 p.m. and I was wondering where Ashley Main, the IRO, was when the doorbell rang. It was him. He was the IRO for both Haylea and Darcy-May and had seen them at their previous reviews. I offered him a drink, but he didn't want one. We went through to the living room, where the buzz of conversation greeted us.

'Have you started without me?' he asked with a smile and sat down. The conversation faded. 'Nice to see you again,' he said to Haylea. 'The last time was at Waysbury.'

Haylea smiled shyly.

'Are we expecting anyone else?' the IRO asked Shari.

'No,' Shari confirmed.

The room was quiet now and Ashley prepared for the meeting by opening his laptop. I'd sat on one of the dining-room chairs I'd brought in, close to the baby monitor. Not knowing how many were coming, I'd brought in extra chairs.

'So this is your second review,' the IRO said to Haylea. 'As you know, we usually start these meetings by introducing ourselves. I'll go first. I'm Ashley Main, the Independent Reviewing Officer.'

'Joy Philips, supervising social worker,' she said.

And so we went round the room, stating our names and roles as the IRO minuted who was present on his laptop.

'Thank you all for coming,' he said as we finished. 'Haylea, this review is about you, and a lot has happened since I last saw you. Would you like to start by telling us how you are and what it's like living here?'

'It's nice, I like it here,' Haylea said, shyly. 'I asked to come here.'

'I know. Darcy-May is here too,' Ashley said, glancing around as if looking for her.

'She's in her cot upstairs,' I said. 'I'll bring her down when she wakes.'

'Ah yes, I can see the baby monitor,' Ashley said, spotting it.

He returned his attention to Haylea. 'So how are you finding it living here with Darcy-May? I must say I had some concerns when I first heard of the arrangement.'

Everyone was looking at Haylea now. 'It's not a problem,' she said. 'I just ignore her.'

'And that works?' the IRO asked, slightly sceptically.

'Yes, I pretend she's not there, like I used to when bad things were happening to me.'

Which summed it up, but what would happen when Haylea could no longer pretend? I wondered. How would she cope with the harsh reality of everything that had happened to her? I couldn't begin to imagine.

CHAPTER EIGHTEEN

A HEAVY HEART

The IRO asked Haylea what she liked about living with me and she said lots of things. 'I like Cathy and her family, and I like this house.'

'So you feel comfortable here?' the IRO said as he typed.

'Yes.'

'What do you do in your spare time?'

'I watch television, and help Cathy bake cakes. Sometimes we go on family outings.'

'That sounds nice. Do you help look after the baby?' the IRO asked, looking up.

'No,' Haylea replied awkwardly.

'I don't ever ask her to,' I said.

The IRO nodded and spoke to Haylea again. 'Thank you for completing your review form. I have read it. Are you happy with the decisions that are being made for you?' It was a standard question asked at reviews, and Haylea nodded.

'And what about your health? Are you well?'

'Yes.'

'Are your optician's and dental check-ups up to date?'

'Yes, they took me when I was at Waysbury,' Haylea confirmed.

'No accidents or serious illnesses since your last review?' It was another standard question.

'No,' Haylea replied.

The review wouldn't go into details about Haylea's past and present health concerns; for example, her pregnancy, the birth of her baby, sexually transmitted diseases and the suggestion that she had been damaged by abuse. It would have been embarrassing for her, and those present who needed to know would have been informed.

'Are you having any contact with your family?' the IRO asked.

'No,' Haylea replied.

'Are you seeing your friends? At your last review you were making friends with some of the others who lived at Waysbury.'

'Not really,' Haylea said. 'No one kept in touch. Cathy said when I go to school I'll make new friends.'

'I'm sure you will,' the IRO agreed with a smile. 'What's happening about school?' He glanced at Jasmine.

'We have found a school that can take Haylea in the new term,' Jasmine replied. 'I'll talk about it when I give my report.'

'Thank you,' the IRO said. But Haylea looked worried and I knew it was going to be a big step for her to get back into the routine of school.

The IRO finished typing and looked at Haylea again. 'I expect you remember from last time that I have to include here if you have been in trouble with the police. Have you?'

'No.'

'And no unauthorized overnight absences? You haven't run away?'

'No. I wouldn't do that. I like it here.'

Joy threw me an appreciative look.

'Excellent,' the IRO said. 'Thank you, Haylea. That's all my questions. Is there anything you would like to say or ask this review?'

'Yes. Does my father know I'm here?'

'No,' Shari said. 'He wasn't given the details, although he wanted them.' Which made me feel slightly uneasy, but Haylea appeared relieved.

I was asked to speak next and I'd just begun by saying that Haylea was a lovely person when Darcy-May began babbling through the monitor. Everyone smiled except Haylea, who as usual managed to block her out. Now Darcy-May was awake I knew it wouldn't be long before she began crying, wanting to be up.

'Would you mind if I brought Darcy-May down first?' I asked the IRO.

'No, of course not. You fetch her.'

I left the room and went quickly upstairs and into my bedroom. Darcy-May grinned and gurgled. I picked her up, kissed her cheek, checked her nappy didn't need changing, and then went downstairs, stopping off at the kitchen on the way to grab a bottle of formula.

As I returned to my chair in the living room everyone looked at Darcy-May and made endearing noises and comments, except of course Haylea, who was staring out of the window.

'She's grown!' the IRO exclaimed. It was three months since he'd seen her at her first review.

'Yes, she's doing very well,' I said.

'She's cute,' Jasmine said, waving at her from across the room.

'Very,' I agreed.

'Coochy-coo,' Joy said, leaning closer to make eye contact.

'She's a lovely baby,' the IRO said. 'And we've got Darcy-May's review after this one. So let's continue and hear from Cathy how well Haylea is doing.'

With Darcy-May in my arms and sucking contentedly on the bottle, I said that Haylea had settled in and was getting on well with my family. 'Haylea has a good appetite and self-care skills,' I continued. 'She likes a long bath in the morning. Unfortunately, she hasn't been sleeping well and tells me she often lies awake at night. Last night she had a nightmare.'

'What about?' the IRO asked, glancing at Haylea.

Haylea didn't answer.

'The abuse she suffered at the hands of her father and others,' I replied.

The IRO had stopped typing and was looking at Haylea with compassion. 'Are you going for counselling?'

Haylea nodded.

'I understand that Haylea has been going, but struggles to talk to the therapist,' I said. 'Hopefully that will improve now.'

'How often do you go?' the IRO asked Haylea.

'Once a week,' she replied.

'It was cancelled this week because the therapist is on holiday,' I added.

'She's sent a report for the review,' Shari said.

'Yes, I saw it, thank you,' the IRO said. Then to Haylea, 'So you want to keep going to these sessions?'

'Yes,' Haylea said.

'The sessions have been during the day,' I said. 'But once Haylea starts school, can they be changed to after school?'

'Yes,' Shari said, and made a note.

I continued by talking about Haylea's routine as the review would expect me to, and said she had enjoyed days out to parks, the zoo and places of interest. 'She can be shy and uncomfortable meeting anyone new or trying new experiences,' I said. 'But she is getting better. I feel she trusts me and I was pleased she felt able to disclose what had happened to her.' I could have said more about Haylea's fragile emotional state and my concerns about how she was able to block out Darcy-May as though she didn't exist, but I'd made Shari and Joy aware of this and it wasn't appropriate to discuss it now in front of Haylea.

'Thank you,' the IRO said. 'Hopefully therapy will help. And Haylea can stay with you until she leaves care?'

'Yes,' I said.

'No complaints from anyone?' he asked. The IRO always asked this at a review.

Those present either said no or shook their head.

'Thank you, Cathy. Let's hear from Haylea's social worker now.' He looked at Shari. 'I think you have a lot to tell us.'

I relaxed a little and Darcy-May finished her bottle.

'Yes, indeed,' Shari said. 'Following what Haylea was able to tell the police, they went to Haylea's father's house and also the address Haylea gave to them. They searched both properties and took away a lot of material. As a result, both men were arrested this morning. They also went to the home of the niece and nephew of the man who lived at the house and they have been taken into care.'

'Thank goodness,' I said with a huge sigh of relief. I assumed these were the children Shari and Joy had spoken of when they'd first arrived. It seemed they *were* related to the man who'd given those disgusting 'parties' and weren't simply calling him 'Uncle' as had been suggested. 'Well done, Haylea,' I said.

She smiled. The others were smiling too. That may seem strange considering the circumstances, but there was a feeling of immense relief in the room. Thanks to Haylea's courage, two evil abusers had been arrested and were no longer at large to harm others. It was also the first step to getting justice for Haylea and the other victims.

'The police seized a lot of material from both houses, which is being examined now,' Shari said. 'I'll know more later.'

'What sort of material?' Jasmine asked. Working in education, she wouldn't necessarily be familiar with the situations that social workers (and foster carers) have to deal with.

'Cameras, webcams, laptops, storage devices, that sort of thing,' Shari said. 'It seems they might have been filming the abuse for some time.'

'Oh my god!' Jasmine cried, visibly shaken. 'I spoke to Mr Walsh on the phone before Haylea came into care when I was trying to get her back into school. How disgusting.'

I looked at Haylea, but she'd gone to that far-away place again that gave her some protection from the present.

'A police interview has been arranged for Haylea tomorrow,' Shari said.

'What time?' I asked. 'I have to take Darcy-May for her vaccination at ten o'clock.'

'It's ten-thirty, but I'll take her,' Shari said.

I nodded and made a note. Joy was also taking notes and the IRO typed.

'That's all I know at present,' Shari said. 'I'll expect to hear more in a few days.'

'Thank you,' the IRO said. Then to Haylea, 'Is there anything you want to ask your social worker about what she's said?'

Haylea returned to the present and shook her head. The IRO looked to Shari to continue. She glanced at her handwritten notes. Her laptop was on her knees in case she wanted to refer to it.

'I'm in touch with the hospital and waiting for the doctor's report,' Shari said. 'Haylea doesn't want another medical so I am hoping it won't be necessary. On another matter, there was an incident involving a member of staff at Waysbury who has been inappropriately texting Haylea and Cathy, but it has been dealt with by the manager Fran Pacton. I understand there were already some concerns about her.' Which was news to me.

'Fran has sent a short report for this review,' the IRO said. 'It covers Haylea's stay there and the reasons for her leaving. I won't read it out unless anyone wants me to.'

No one did, so Shari began winding up her report to the review. 'The care plan remains unchanged and overall Haylea has been doing very well in placement here. I think the routine of school will help her too. She's promised me she will try to share more with her therapist when the sessions resume next week.'

'Thank you,' the IRO said. 'What happened about the home tutoring? I see it was mentioned at Haylea's last review.'

'The funding came through but after the schools broke up. Home tutors only work term time and Haylea will be in mainstream school next term.'

'So it didn't happen,' the IRO said as he typed. 'Anything else?'

'Not at present,' Shari confirmed.

'Joy, would you like to add anything?' the IRO asked my SSW.

'Yes, I'm in regular contact with Cathy and as one of our very experienced foster carers I know she is giving Haylea a good standard of care. She will ask for help if necessary and keeps me updated.'

'Thank you. So no complaints?'

'None.'

'Jasmine, would you like to go next?'

Jasmine opened her laptop and, looking at Haylea, said, 'You've missed rather a lot of school in the past for various reasons and I know you don't want to miss any more. The school I've found is ideal. It's small, with a very good support system. Turnbridge. Do you know it?'

Haylea shook her head. I knew of the school, although I hadn't had any children go there.

'I had a meeting with the Head and she's offered you a place to start in September. I know the school from placing other young people there. It's excellent. Ideal for you. You can have a look at their website. It includes details of term dates, school uniform, their policy, clubs and activities and so forth.'

'That sounds good, thank you,' the IRO said. We were all looking at Haylea for her reaction. It would need her cooperation to make it work.

'I don't know where it is,' she said, worried. 'Will I have to go on the bus?'

'Not until you feel comfortable going on the bus,' Shari said. 'I'm sure Cathy can take and collect you to begin with.'

'Yes,' I said. 'Also, we'll go over during the holidays to take a look from the outside.' I'd done this with other children who were starting a new school and it seemed to help. 'We've got plenty of time,' I said. 'We could also do a dummy run on the bus. I think it's about half an hour's bus journey. I'm sure the 152 goes straight there from the High Street, but we'll sort that out. Don't worry.'

'Thank you,' Haylea said doubtfully. 'I don't want to get lost.'

'You won't,' I replied.

The IRO smiled encouragingly, but I knew it wasn't just the journey that was worrying Haylea; it was the whole concept of going to school after so long away from the routine. Thankfully I had a month to prepare her.

Jasmine said a little bit more about the school, emphasizing its attributes and how appropriate it was for Haylea. Their uniform was grey trousers or skirt with a maroon jumper – details of where to buy the uniform were on their website.

'Thank you, Jasmine,' the IRO said as she finished. 'That's most helpful.' He concentrated on his laptop for a few moments and then looked at Haylea. 'Your therapist has sent a report, but I won't read it out. There is a suggestion that you might be happier with a different therapist when one becomes available.'

'No, it's fine,' Haylea said. 'I just couldn't tell her what had happened, but I'll talk to her in future, I promise.'

'OK,' the IRO said gently. 'It's not compulsory. It's to help you.'

'I know. I will go.'

The IRO made a note and asked if anyone else had anything to say. They didn't, so he set the date for the next review in three months' time and closed the meeting by saying, 'Good luck in your new school, Haylea. I am sure you will do very well.'

'So am I,' Jasmine said, and stood to leave.

Jasmine was the only one not needed at Darcy-May's review, which was following straight on from Haylea's. Darcy-May was now asleep in my arms, so I laid her in the bouncing cradle and then saw Jasmine out.

'I'll be in touch,' she said at the door. 'But if you or Haylea have any questions, phone me.'

'Thank you.' I think Jasmine appreciated just what a big step this was going to be for Haylea.

As I closed the front door Haylea appeared in the hall. 'I don't have to stay for the next review, do I?' she asked.

'No, love. It's up to you.'

'I'll be in my room,' she said, and went upstairs.

I returned to the living room and offered everyone a drink. There were ten minutes to go before Darcy-May's review began.

'A tea would be welcome,' the IRO said. 'I understand we're just waiting for Nia to arrive from the Family Finding team.'

'Yes, that's right,' Shari confirmed. 'A good match has been found for Darcy-May and I've asked Nia here to bring us up to date. I'll have a tea too, please, Cathy.'

Joy asked for a glass of water and I left the room to make the drinks with a heavy heart. While it was important for Darcy-May to be with her forever family as soon as possible, in so doing she would be leaving my family. As a foster carer I know I'm likely to have to say good-bye to the child at some point, but that doesn't make it any easier.

CHAPTER NINETEEN

TELL THE POLICE

Once Nia, the social worker from the Family Finding team, had arrived, the IRO opened Darcy-May's review by asking us to introduce ourselves. When we'd finished he said, 'Isn't Haylea going to join us then?'

'No,' I confirmed.

'I suppose that's understandable,' the IRO said, and made a note.

'Where is she?' Shari asked me.

'Upstairs in her room.'

'I'll see her before I go.'

I was asked to speak first and I began by saying what a joy it was to look after Darcy-May, then I described her feeding and sleeping routine, our visits to the clinic where she was weighed and measured, her development, and so forth. It was easy finding lots of positive things to say about her. 'She's such a happy and contented baby,' I enthused. 'Her adoptive parents are very lucky to be having her. She's a treasure.'

'You're going to miss her when she goes,' Joy said.

'Yes, very much.'

'Although I expect it will be easier for you just having Haylea,' the IRO added.

'It will certainly be different,' I said. 'I'm not sure about easier.'

'How is Haylea?' the IRO asked, looking up from his laptop.

'She seems to be coping, just,' I said honestly. 'I think it's a release for her now she's finally started talking about the abuse. But goodness knows how she will ever come to terms with what's happened.'

'No, indeed,' the IRO agreed. 'I was surprised she felt up to attending her review. She did well. How is she with Darcy-May?'

'She completely ignores her,' I said. 'She can shut her out as if she doesn't exist, even when they're in the same room or the car.'

'So Haylea never feeds her or plays with her?' Nia asked. She had a notepad open on her lap.

'No, not at all. She never has. I haven't encouraged her as I knew the care plan was for Darcy-May to go for adoption.'

'So there is no bond between them?' Nia asked. 'It's something adoptive parents usually want to know.'

'None as far as I can see. I mean, Haylea must be aware that Darcy-May is hers, but she can block her out, just as she blocked out the abuse – that's what she told me.'

'That's sad,' Nia said, making a note.

Everyone was looking at Darcy-May still sleeping peacefully in the bouncing cradle.

'I assume Haylea's therapist will help her address this in counselling?' the IRO said to Shari.

'I assume so.'

'Cathy, please continue,' the IRO said. 'You mentioned a vaccination tomorrow.'

'Yes, Darcy-May will be having the last of the six-in-one vaccine tomorrow. I'm pleased to say there are no more after that until she is a year old.'

'What does the six-in-one protect against?' Nia asked.

'I'll have to check,' I said, and reached for the Red Book, which was on the floor beside me with my fostering folder. I opened it and flicked through to the relevant page. 'Hepatitis B, diphtheria, Hib, which is a type of flu, polio, tetanus and whooping cough.'

'Thank you,' Nia said as she wrote.

'Her Red Book is up to date and I'll pass it on to the adoptive parents,' I added.

'Do you have any other material for the adopters?' Nia asked.

'I'm keeping up a Life Story Book,' I said. 'Is that what you mean?'

'Yes. Great.'

'So Darcy-May is healthy?' the IRO said, going through the questions the review needed to cover.

'Yes, absolutely.'

'I see from the last review that the health visitor was present, but she's not here today.'

'I didn't ask her,' Shari said. 'Cathy visits the clinic regularly and sees a health visitor there. It's usual when a baby is this age.'

'OK, thank you,' the IRO said as he typed. 'Anything else you want to add?' he asked me.

'I don't think so. Darcy-May is meeting all the developmental milestones and is a lovely baby.' Again, everyone looked at her.

The IRO asked Shari to give her report and she began by confirming the care plan was up to date and Darcy-

May would remain with me and then be placed with her adoptive family. 'Nia will tell us more about them shortly,' Shari said. 'But given Haylea's recent disclosures about abuse, it's probable that Darcy-May is the result of rape by one of her abusers or even incest by her father. I shall talk to Haylea tomorrow when I take her for the police interview about having a DNA test done to establish paternity.'

'That would be useful,' Nia said. 'Adoptive parents usually want to know as much as possible about the baby's history.'

'What do they know at present?' Joy asked.

'Only that Darcy-May was born to a teenage mother who made the decision straight away that she should go for adoption.'

'That decision makes more sense now we know how Darcy-May was conceived,' the IRO said sombrely.

'Yes,' I agreed. 'I have wondered if the baby looks like Haylea's abuser, and that's the reason she can't bear to look at her.'

I saw Nia grimace. It was a horrific thought.

'It's possible,' the IRO agreed. 'Will Haylea be offered contact with Darcy-May after she is placed for adoption?' she asked Shari.

'Just letterbox if she wants it,' Shari replied. 'Haylea will be able to send birthday and Christmas cards via the social services and write a letter to go in them if she wishes. The adoptive parents will send an annual report on how Darcy-May is doing for Haylea. That also comes through us.'

'Do you think she will want to have letterbox contact?' Nia asked me.

'Not a present, but I suppose it could change in the future.'

'So the adoptive parents you have in mind don't know the circumstances in which Darcy-May was conceived?' Joy asked Nia.

'No, I only found out just now. I will tell them when I see them on Friday.'

Shari continued by saying that if all went to plan then Darcy-May would be with her adoptive parents in three to six months' time. I swallowed hard. Nia was then asked to speak.

'I have another meeting on Friday with the adoptive parents,' she said brightly, sitting upright. 'Cathy, I'd like you to come so you can tell the couple all about Darcy-May. They are so looking forward to meeting you. I emailed you the details before I came here today, and to you, Joy.' While it was usual for the prospective adoptive parents to meet the foster carer at this stage, I could have done with a bit more notice. I would have to make provision for Darcy-May and Haylea. Joy was looking thoughtfully at her diary too.

'It's at eleven o'clock at the council offices,' Nia continued, addressing me. 'Please bring Darcy-May's Life Story Book and any other material you have to share with them.'

'I assume you don't want me to bring Darcy-May?' I said, making a note of the time in my diary. I'd read her email later.

'No, not until we start the introductions, which won't be until after we've been to panel.'

'I'll need to arrange childcare for her and Haylea,' I said.

'Fine,' Nia said, apparently not appreciating that wasn't going to be so easy at very short notice. She continued to talk about the prospective adopters – Jessica and Andrew, a married couple in their early thirties who couldn't have children of their own. They lived eighty miles away – Family Finding often covers the whole country. 'They both work full time,' Nia said. 'But Jessica's employer is aware that she will be leaving work to become a full-time mother as soon as their baby arrives. Jessica and Andrew are a very good match for Darcy-May, physically and culturally. They will be able to provide an excellent standard of living for her.'

The IRO nodded as he typed.

'They are already approved to adopt,' Nia continued, her enthusiasm palpable. 'So I'll be taking them to the next matching panel, then we can start the introductions. I love this bit. It's so rewarding.'

'They're a very good match,' Shari confirmed. She would have seen their details and had possibly already met them.

'Jessica and Andrew are only children,' Nia said. 'Both sets of parents are alive, so Darcy-May will have lots of grandparents to spoil her. I've met them and they are so looking forward to the arrival of their first grandchild.'

As Nia continued expounding the virtues of Jessica and Andrew I heard Haylea creep downstairs and go into the kitchen and pour herself a glass of water. I wondered if she'd changed her mind and would join us, but she went upstairs again. I'd check on her once Darcy-May's review had ended.

Confirming that she'd see Joy and me at the meeting on Friday, Nia wound up what she had to say as positively as she had begun. 'I know Jessica and Andrew will make excellent parents for Darcy-May.'

'Thank you,' the IRO said, and finished typing. 'Joy, would you like to say anything?'

'Yes, I'd like to thank Cathy for all she's done for Darcy-May. She has clearly flourished in her care. Cathy will do all she can to ensure Darcy-May's move to her permanent family runs smoothly. I'll be at the meeting on Friday as long as I can change the appointment I already have in my diary. I should be able to.' Then, turning to me, she asked, 'Will you need help with child-care?'

'Yes.'

'I'll talk to you about it later.'

The review wouldn't be interested in my childcare arrangements. With no further business, the IRO set the date for Darcy-May's next review in three months' time, thanked us all for coming and closed the meeting.

I left Joy looking after Darcy-May while I saw the IRO and Nia out. I then went to the kitchen for a bottle of formula before returning to the living room.

'Is Haylea still in her bedroom?' Shari asked, standing.

'Yes.'

'I'll go up and see her then.'

'You know where her room is?'

'Yes, thanks.'

As I fed Darcy-May Joy said, 'We have a newly approved foster carer, Mrs Abebe. I'll ask her to babysit for you on Friday.'

'Thank you. It was rather short notice.'

'I know.'

'Do you want her to come here? It will be less disruptive than taking Darcy-May and Haylea to her house.'

'Yes, please.'

'I'll phone her later today and give her your number so you can arrange the time.'

'Thank you,' I said again. I was grateful.

'I'll see myself out,' Joy said and, packing away her notepad and pen, left. I continued feeding Darcy-May.

Shari was with Haylea for about fifteen minutes and then returned to the living room.

'How is she?' I asked.

'Worried about the police interview tomorrow. I've tried to reassure her. I hope she doesn't back out. I'll collect her at ten o'clock and bring her here after. I notice she's still got her birthday cards on display in her room,' Shari added with a sad smile. 'She wanted to show them to me again.'

'I know. I don't think she's ever had cards before. They can stay on show for as long as she wants.'

Having seen Shari out, I carried Darcy-May upstairs and, calling out to Haylea that I was just going to change her, I went into my bedroom and laid her on the changing mat on my bed. A few moments later I heard Haylea come round the landing and then she appeared at my open bedroom door.

'Hi, love, are you OK?' I asked, glancing up from what I was doing.

'Not really,' she said glumly. 'I'm worried about tomorrow.'

'I understand, but the police officers are lovely. They won't put you under any pressure.'

'But they are going to ask me for details about what happened.'

'Yes. I expect they will.'

'But I can't tell them. It's too horrible. There's more stuff that I haven't told you.' Which Haylea had said before.

'I can only guess at the horror you have been through, love. But it is important you tell the police as much as you can so those evil men can be punished.'

'That's what Shari said, but they could be punished if I don't go for the interview. There is other evidence – you know, the videos they took.'

'Yes, but it would help if you could give your evidence. The police will speak to those two other children as well. It all helps to make sure your abusers are convicted and given as long a prison sentence as possible.'

I could see from her face she was still doubtful and I guessed she'd had a similar conversation with Shari. I'd finished changing Darcy-May and I put her in her cot so I could concentrate on Haylea.

'Let's continue this in your room,' I suggested.

I followed Haylea round the landing and into her bedroom where we both sat on the edge of her bed. The room was tidy – it always was: her birthday and leaving cards, a few books and some soft toys she'd bought while we'd been shopping were arranged neatly on the shelves.

'I hate the thought of the police officers seeing those videos of me like that,' Haylea said quietly.

'I know, but it's their job and they are specially trained. Sadly, they will have seen similar before.'

'Do you really think so?'

'Yes,' I said, and took her hand in mine. She didn't take it away.

'They won't think I'm a slut?'

'No, of course not. You are a victim. A child who has been very badly abused.'

'That man – my father,' Haylea said, not wanting to use the term. 'He used to call me a slut. He said I was a dirty little slut who enjoyed being fucked. He thought it was funny. I didn't enjoy it, Cathy. I hate him and the others who did those things to me.' She was close to tears.

I instinctively squeezed her hand.

'I'm sorry,' she said.

'For what? You've got nothing to be sorry for.'

'For upsetting you.'

Tears stung the back of my eyes. Here she was, the victim of shocking abuse, and she was worried about upsetting me.

'I'm all right, love,' I said. 'But you need to tell the police what your father said and did and anything else you can remember. Do you know who the other men were?'

'Some of them were friends of his – my father. I know who they are but not the others. They were at those parties and the room was always dark, and they wore masks or those black balaclavas with just their eyes and mouth showing.'

I struggled to keep my voice even as I pictured the horror of that scene. 'Make sure you tell the police all of this,' I said again. 'I'll tell Shari too. She'll pass it on.' What Haylea was telling me was all evidence, which would hopefully be used to prosecute and convict those responsible.

I could hear Darcy-May beginning to grizzle. She'd had a sleep earlier so I guessed she wouldn't want another one now.

'I'll have to see to Darcy-May in a minute,' I told Haylea.

She nodded.

'Haylea, there is something I'd like to ask you. Something I've been wondering about.'

She looked at me questioningly.

'Does Darcy-May remind you of anyone?'

She gave another small nod.

'Can you tell me who?'

'My father and his brother – my uncle. They look similar.'

'And they both abused you?'

'Yes.'

'This isn't the uncle who gave the parties?'

'No, I'm talking about my uncle. He …' she began but couldn't say any more.

'It's all right, love, but tell the police, please.'

CHAPTER TWENTY

TRAPPED IN A WEB

Haylea spent the rest of the day worrying about the police interview. She kept asking me questions about what was going to happen and the things she might be asked. I reassured her as best I could, but I began to think she might not go, especially when she said, 'I really don't think I can talk to them.'

There weren't any more reassurances I could give her. 'Just do your best,' I said.

She hardly ate anything at dinner and didn't talk at all. Paula asked her what was wrong and Haylea said brusquely, 'Nothing,' then left the table and went to her room.

I told Paula it wasn't her fault and I went upstairs after Haylea, but she said she wanted to be alone, so reluctantly I did as she asked. I just hoped that if she didn't attend the police interview then there was still sufficient evidence to prosecute her abusers. The alternative – that they would be free to continue abusing – was too awful to contemplate.

Haylea spent most of the evening in her bedroom. I went up every so often and tried talking to her, but she said again she wanted to be alone. At eight o'clock I found she had changed into her nightwear and was in bed. She had her earphones in and was listening to music, which I assumed was offering her some distraction from the worry of the interview tomorrow. I told her I was downstairs if she wanted me and she nodded. Darcy-May was in her cot for the night.

A few moments later my mobile rang and a woman with a lovely warm Caribbean accent asked, 'Is that Cathy Glass?'

'Yes.'

'It's Ines Abebe here. I think you're expecting my call. Is this a good time?'

'Perfect,' I said, sitting on the sofa in the living room. 'Thank you for agreeing to look after Haylea and Darcy-May on Friday.'

'You're very welcome. I think Shari told you that my hubby and I have just been approved to foster.'

'Yes, congratulations.'

'Thank you. They want to ease us into it gently by giving us some babysitting first,' she said with a chuckle. 'But, Cathy, I've brought up four children of my own, plus three of my sisters, so I know a bit about raising children.' She laughed again and I found myself smiling.

'They always like to give new carers a bit of respite cover first.'

'I know and I don't mind. So, tell me what I need to know and what time to be there on Friday. I believe you're going to an adoption meeting for the baby you're fostering.'

'Yes, that's right, Darcy-May. I will have to leave here at about ten-thirty so if you could come a bit earlier, say ten-fifteen, I can show you where everything is.'

'That's fine with me. And Darcy-May is four months old, and Haylea is her teenage mother?' Shari would have told her this.

'Yes, although Haylea doesn't participate in the care of the baby. She may want to stay in her bedroom. If she does, please check on her regularly. She's been through a lot.'

Usually when a carer looks after a child on respite the permanent carer sends them some basic details, but this was short notice and I hadn't had time, and I'd only be gone a couple of hours. It would be different if they'd been staying with her for the night.

'Don't you worry, Cathy,' Ines said in her sing-song voice. 'I'll look after the pair of them, just as I did my sister's children.'

'Thank you. That was kind of you to bring up your sister's children. I bet seven kept you on your toes.'

'You're telling me,' she giggled. 'And they were all about the same age. The youngest two are still with me. The rest have flown the nest. My hubby was good, though – hands-on father – not like some you get back home who think childcare is woman's work.'

'Where are you from originally?' I asked.

'Jamaica.'

'Wonderful. I'd love to go there one day.'

'Well, when you do be sure to let me know and I'll give you the address of my family home. It's up in the hills away from it all. There's my brother and another sister there at present. You'd be made very welcome.'

'That is kind of you. Do you manage to go back at all?'

'Yes, every year for three weeks. I told them that when I applied to foster. I said I visit my family for three weeks every November and that can't be changed. I thought it best to get that out of the way at the start. Nothing stops me from seeing my family.'

'Good for you.'

We continued talking and one subject led to another so that we were on the phone for nearly an hour. Ines was someone I immediately warmed to and gelled with – a naturally friendly person. Eventually I told her what she needed to know about Haylea and Darcy-May for Friday and we said goodbye. Afterwards, I felt better for talking to her, just as I used to with my mother, although Ines would be my age, possibly younger.

I checked on Haylea and she still had her earpieces in so I hoped that listening to music was giving her some distraction from her worries. I returned downstairs and, with a mug of tea, sat at my computer, where I updated my log and then emailed Shari, including what Haylea had said that evening.

Before I went to bed I checked on Haylea again and she was still listening to music.

'Can I keep my phone on for a while?' she asked.

'Yes, but try to get some sleep.'

'I will,' she said.

'Goodnight, love.'

I came out of her room, hoping she'd find the courage to attend the police interview tomorrow. I'd looked after children before who'd been severely abused and had been interviewed by the police. While they'd been very worried before, once they'd gone they felt better for it and were pleased they'd done it. Just to be able to tell the police can be cathartic.

* * *

That night Haylea had a terrifying nightmare that sent fear through me too. She woke in the early hours, screaming hysterically. I was straight out of bed and rushed round the landing into her bedroom. The light was on, as she'd left it, and Haylea was sitting up in bed, eyes closed, screaming and trying to pull something from her face and head. There were strands of hair between her fingers that had come out. 'Get off! I can't breathe!' she cried.

'Haylea, it's Cathy. You're dreaming. Stop it.' I took her hands from her face and held them tight as she tried to pull at her hair again. She was hot and gasping for breath.

'No, let me go!' she screamed, eyes still shut.

'Haylea, it's Cathy.'

I heard Paula's bedroom door open and Darcy-May start to cry.

Paula looked in, as shocked as I was. 'Can you settle Darcy-May?' I said, still battling with Haylea. 'Give her a bottle if necessary.'

Worried, she went to do as I'd asked. Haylea was still clawing at whatever she thought was covering her face and head. 'Haylea. Open your eyes. You're having a nightmare. It's not real.'

I held onto her hands, restraining her so she wouldn't do herself more harm. She was strong and kept trying to get away. 'You're having a bad dream. Open your eyes!' I cried loudly. And finally she did.

She stared distractedly around the room. 'Haylea, you've had a dream,' I said again. 'Haylea?'

She looked at me, terror in her eyes. The dream hadn't gone yet.

'Haylea, it's me, Cathy. You had a nightmare. You're safe now.'

'Where am I?' she asked, bewildered.

'In your bedroom, at home with me. You've had a nightmare, you're safe.'

Her hands began to relax and gradually her breathing regulated. I let go of them and she gingerly touched and patted her face as if feeling for something. 'It's gone,' she said. 'It's not there.'

'That's right. You had a bad dream.'

'Oh Cathy, it was awful. It was so real. I was trapped in a spider's web. I could feel its sticky threads criss-crossing all over my face and head like glue. I couldn't open my mouth or breathe. I was trapped and couldn't move, then a giant spider began coming towards me. I could see its eyes and arched legs. I couldn't move and I knew that when he got to me he was going to eat me alive.'

She grabbed my hand and it was all I could do to stop myself from crying out too. 'You're safe,' I said again.

'It was so real. I could feel its sticky web.' She shivered. 'I kept struggling, but I couldn't break free. Thank goodness you saved me.'

She allowed me to put my arm around her shoulders and I comforted her.

I hate spiders and I was unsettled by the graphic image of her nightmare, although it didn't take much to see where it had come from. Trapped in a sticky web and at the mercy of an advancing predator. Haylea had spent most of her life trapped in an evil web of paedophiles, at their mercy and waiting to be devoured by them. I felt the full horror of her dream.

I sat with Haylea until she was able to go back to sleep. During that time Paula fed Darcy-May and then returned to her own room. Once I could leave Haylea, I went to my room where Darcy-May was asleep again in her cot. I would thank Paula in the morning rather than disturb her now.

It was nearly 3.30 a.m. when I got back into bed but I didn't go to sleep. I was shaken by Haylea's dream and could picture only too clearly the terror of what she'd described. I lay awake listening to Darcy-May's gentle breathing and her occasional snuffles. Thankfully she was safe from the horror of what had been her mother's life. But it could have been very different, I thought with renewed horror, if she'd gone home as Haylea's father had wanted. My stomach churned. I knew from my foster-carer training that some paedophiles abused babies, and others watched the abuse online. This type of material is hidden on what's called the dark web, and as fast as one website is closed another one opens. It was possible that Haylea's abuse was already out there.

I must have dropped off to sleep at some point for it was 7.15 when I woke. Darcy-May, topped up from the bottle Paula had given her, was still asleep. I could hear Paula moving in her room. I went round and thanked her for her help during the night and then left her to get ready for work. I looked in on Haylea and she was asleep too, so I quietly closed her bedroom door. She didn't have to get up yet.

Once I'd showered and dressed, I felt a bit better, although the horror of Haylea's dream stayed with me. It was 8.30 before Haylea got up. She came downstairs in her nightwear. I was in the living room with Darcy-May. Paula had left for work.

'How are you?' I asked.

'Tired,' she said, rubbing her eyes.

'I'm not surprised. Do you remember your dream?'

'Yes, but I'm trying not to.'

I changed the subject. 'Let's get you some breakfast and then you need to get ready for when Shari arrives at ten o'clock. I'll be thinking of you while I'm at the clinic. Darcy-May is having a vaccination this morning.'

'I think I'd rather have that,' Haylea said, grimacing, and came with me into the kitchen.

I sat Darcy-May in her bouncing cradle and suggested to Haylea that she had a cooked breakfast as she hadn't had much to eat the evening before, but she just wanted cornflakes with milk, and a glass of juice.

'How long do you think I will be there?' she asked as we sat at the table. I took her question as a promising sign she was going to attend the police interview.

'I don't know exactly,' I replied. 'A couple of hours. It rather depends on how much you can tell them.'

'What shall I wear?' she asked as she ate.

'One of your dresses maybe?' I suggested. 'It's going to be warm again today. They're smart and you don't wear them very often now.'

'Do I have to wear one of those?' she asked.

'No. It was just an idea.'

'I think I'll wear something you bought me and get rid of those dresses.'

'That's fine. We can pack them away.' I'd bought Haylea clothes since she'd been living with me, when we'd gone shopping together. They were fashionable clothes more suitable for a teenager.

'I don't like those dresses,' she said.

'No, all right. Our tastes change.'

'He – my father – always made me wear dresses like that,' Haylea said, her voice flat. 'He said he didn't want me wearing what other teenagers wore because they looked like sluts.'

I remembered Fran had told me that when a member of staff at Waysbury had taken Haylea shopping she'd chosen long dresses for 'modesty'. It was now clear they hadn't been her choice but the lingering control of her father.

'He said the only place I could be a slut was at home with him,' Haylea continued. 'He bought me other clothes, and make-up, that I had to wear in the house with just him. Not like the dresses I wore outside, but sexy. He said I should be a sexy slut at home with him.'

Haylea had said this in a matter-of-fact tone, while I was appalled, but then she'd had to live with his abuse for all those years. 'Make sure you tell the police that,' was all I said.

I sat with Haylea while she finished her breakfast, then, when she went upstairs to dress, I packed the baby bag ready to go to the clinic later. Once Haylea was ready, she came down and we sat in the living room talking generally while we waited for Shari. Darcy-May was in her bouncing cradle making cute baby noises, which as usual Haylea ignored. She talked about her new school, which she would start in the new term in September. She'd already looked at their website. I said I'd take her in the car to see exactly where it was. She talked about the weather and having another family outing. Unlike the previous day, she didn't mention the police interview at all. I suspected she'd hived it off, as she had done with other traumas she'd faced in life, in order to survive.

When the doorbell rang at 10 a.m. Haylea came with me to answer it.

'Hi, all set?' Shari asked brightly.

'Yes,' I replied as Haylea slipped on her shoes. Shari looked relieved.

'I got your email, thank you,' Shari said to me. 'I'll pass it on.'

Haylea left the house in silence.

'Good luck!' I called after her.

She threw me a weak smile and then got into the car. I watched it pull away, then I went indoors where I collected Darcy-May and the baby bag and left to go to the clinic.

As with her previous vaccinations, Darcy-May cried as the needle went in but quickly recovered. My thoughts immediately returned to Haylea and how she was getting on at the police station, and they stayed with her as the morning passed. I made lunch, played with Darcy-May and then settled her in the cot for an afternoon nap, which allowed me to work at my computer. I knew that the police would do all they could to encourage Haylea to tell them what she knew, but if she couldn't there would be a cut-off point when they would terminate the interview so she wasn't put under pressure. I was expecting her home any time now, but it was 2.30 before she arrived.

'She's done very well,' Shari said. 'We've only just finished.' Haylea came quietly into the hall.

'Well done,' I said to her as she took off her shoes.

'I'm going to get a drink,' she said, and disappeared down the hall.

'Are you coming in?' I asked Shari.

'No, I have another meeting shortly. But we're all very pleased with Haylea. The police have enough evidence to search the homes of others they think were involved. Unfortunately, Haylea asked them where her father and that other man were now and the officer had to tell her they'd been released on bail. She's very worried that they will come looking for her. I've told her they don't know where she is, and the police told her if she did see either of them around here to tell you or phone the police straight away. One of the conditions of their bail is that they can't go anywhere near Haylea or those other two children.'

'I'll tell her again,' I said. 'Although she never goes out without me anyway.'

'Good. They're unlikely to be stupid enough to break their bail conditions and try to approach her. They know they'll be straight back into custody if they do.'

So neither of us were unduly worried and Shari said goodbye and left. I was aware it was usual for suspects to be released on bail pending further investigations or their trial, so I reassured Haylea. As Shari had said, they wouldn't be stupid and break their bail condition and risk going straight to prison. Would they?

CHAPTER TWENTY-ONE

AN INNOCENT BABY

Now the ordeal of the police interview was behind her Haylea said she was hungry, so I made her a fry-up – an all-day breakfast – egg, bacon, beans, tomatoes and toast. She could have cooked it herself, but I liked to mother her. She'd had no real mothering in the past. She ate the lot and then said she was going to sort through her clothes and get rid of those her father had bought for her. If I'd had any idea of the connotations attached to those long matronly dresses, I would have suggested clearing them out sooner. But Haylea had only recently started talking about what had happened to her, so I'd assumed, as they had at Waysbury, that her clothes were her choice.

I gave her some plastic bin bags and asked if she wanted any help, but she didn't. Half an hour later she came down with two bin bags stuffed full of clothes.

'Shall I put them outside in the dustbin?' she asked.

'No. I'd better keep them for now until Shari has a chance to offer those your father bought back to him.'

'Why?' Haylea asked, astonished.

'Because they are legally his. It's the same with any child who comes into care,' I explained. 'The child's belongings that came from home are offered back to the parents before they are disposed of.'

She pulled a face.

'I know. I'll put them away and let Shari know,' I said, and took them from her.

'Then can I throw them out?' she asked.

'Yes, or we could take them to the charity shop in the High Street.'

I put the bags of clothes out of sight at the back of the cupboard under the stairs. Haylea asked if we could bake cakes together, so with Darcy-May watching from her bouncing cradle we made cupcakes. Then we prepared dinner for when Paula arrived home from work. There was a much better atmosphere at the table that evening than the day before when Haylea had been very worried about going for the police interview. She talked and told Paula of her day and then asked her about hers, which was kind.

During the evening, while Paula was in her bedroom relaxing after a busy day at work, I explained to Haylea that another foster carer, Ines, was coming tomorrow to stay with her and Darcy-May while I went to an adoption meeting. 'She sounded really nice on the phone,' I said. 'But you get on with whatever you want to do. She will look after Darcy-May.'

'Is that because I don't?' Haylea asked.

'Partly. Then on Saturday,' I continued brightly, 'we've got Emma's first birthday party.'

Haylea's face clouded over.

'What's the matter? It will be fun.'

'I know. It's just me being silly. The word "party". Don't worry, I'll get over it.'

'Yes, of course,' I said, realizing. But it was likely to be a long time before Haylea could hear the word 'party' without associating it with the atrocities committed at that man's house.

'I haven't got Emma anything for her birthday,' Haylea then said.

'Don't worry, I've got plenty to give her from all of us.'

'But I'd like to buy her a card and present of my own. Could we go to the shops tomorrow afternoon when you get back?'

'Yes.'

'You'll come with me?'

'I will.'

That night I heard Haylea get up to use the toilet. I'm a light sleeper from years of listening out for children. I then heard her moving around her room, so I went to see if she was all right. It was 1.30 a.m. I knocked lightly on her bedroom door and opened it a little. The light was on low and she was just getting back into bed.

'Are you OK?' I asked quietly.

'Yes, but I can't sleep. Can I listen to music on my phone?'

'Yes.' I smiled and came out.

Haylea was sensible and not one to phone or text friends all night. Indeed, she hardly knew anyone. So if listening to music helped her relax that was fine with me.

I didn't hear her again during the night, and the following morning when she was up, dressed and having her breakfast, I asked her what sort of music she liked.

'I listen to all sorts, but at night I listen to classical music. It's soothing and helps me go to sleep.'

I nodded, impressed.

'Cook used to tell me to count sheep if I couldn't sleep,' Haylea said. 'But their bleating kept me awake.'

It was a moment before I realized she was joking. We both laughed, and not for the first time I thought what an amazing person Haylea was. Despite all she'd been through, she had managed to retain a sense of humour and could be witty. I truly admired her tenacity.

'Where does a sheep get its hair cut?' I asked.

'The baa-baa's,' she replied, and we laughed again.

Ines arrived just after ten o'clock and was as bright and bubbly in person as she had sounded on the phone. I'd answered the front door with Darcy-May in my arms.

'Aren't you the most adorable baby ever,' Ines said, chucking her under the chin.

Some babies cry when meeting anyone new, but Darcy-May was used to it and gurgled and grinned, which pleased Ines.

'She likes me,' Ines said.

'She does,' I agreed. Although I thought it would be impossible not to like Ines. A big lady with a big heart, she had a natural warmth and beauty. She was wearing a gaily patterned yellow-and-orange summer dress, which reflected her outgoing personality.

'Come and meet Haylea,' I said, and led the way down the hall and into the living room. I'd already told Ines on the phone what she needed to know about Haylea, including that she was often wary of those she didn't know.

'Hello, love, how are you?' Ines asked with a smile.

'OK,' Haylea replied guardedly. 'I'm going to my room.'

'All right, love. I'll be down here if you need me,' Ines replied easily, and threw me a knowing look.

With Darcy-May still in my arms, I showed Ines into the kitchen and where the bottles of formula, tea, coffee, cakes and biscuits were. 'Help yourself to whatever you fancy,' I said.

'Don't tempt me,' she replied. 'Those chocolate digestives are my favourite.'

I then took Ines upstairs to my bedroom where the baby mat, nappies and creams were. 'Darcy-May doesn't usually have a nap in her cot until after lunch,' I said. 'I should be back by then, but she often takes short naps downstairs in the bouncing cradle, on the sofa or on my lap.'

'I'll remember,' Ines said. 'Will she come to me?'

I passed Darcy-May to her and she snuggled against her chest.

'No problem,' I said. 'If you'd like to take her downstairs, I'll say goodbye to Haylea.'

Haylea's bedroom door was slightly ajar so I poked my head round.

'I'm off now, love. See you in a couple of hours. I'll make us lunch when I get back, but if you're hungry you can make yourself a sandwich. Offer Ines one too.'

Haylea nodded. I came out, leaving her door slightly open, and went downstairs. Ines was in the living room with Darcy-May on her lap. I checked she had everything she needed and then, saying goodbye, left. I had Darcy-May's Life Story Book tucked under my arm and her Red Book, and a USB stick containing more photos and video clips of her in my bag. The main purpose of today's meeting was so that Andrew and Jessica could hear all about Darcy-May first-hand from me. They would have received basic details when they were first matched with her. Now I would bring them up to date, and personalize it by talking about her development, routine and the myriad of little details that made her who she was and such a treasure. Although I was sad to be losing Darcy-May, I needed to be professional and do the next bit of my job as a foster carer, to make the transition to her forever family run smoothly.

I parked close to the council offices, went into the building and registered at reception. As I was hanging my ID pass around my neck Joy joined me. I waited for her to register and then we went upstairs together to the first floor.

'Exciting day for Jessica and Andrew,' she remarked as we went.

'Absolutely,' I agreed. 'I've got plenty of material to show them.'

'Great.'

We found the meeting room and Joy gave a brief knock on the door as we went in. Shari, Nia and a smartly dressed couple in their thirties who I took to be the prospective adopters were already seated at the table in the centre of the room.

'We're not late, I hope,' Joy said, voicing my thoughts.

'No, I asked Jessica and Andrew to meet us early,' Nia replied rather formally.

I smiled at the couple as I sat down, but they didn't return my smile. Indeed, they looked very serious, even slightly angry, and I wondered why.

I set the Life Story Book on the table, pulled in my chair and waited. Joy was looking expectantly at Shari, who would normally have opened the meeting. 'Shall we start with introductions?' Joy asked, after a moment.

'Yes, go ahead,' Shari said.

'I'm Joy Philips, Cathy's supervising social worker,' she said, looking at the couple.

'Cathy Glass, Darcy-May's foster carer,' I said, with another smile.

'Andrew and Jessica Beard,' he said stiffly, introducing them both.

'Nia Page, Family Finding team,' she said, and took her laptop from her bag.

'Shari Drew, social worker for Darcy-May. I'll take a few notes of the meeting.' She opened a flip-pad on the desk in front of her, then paused, apparently uncertain what to say next. 'I invited everyone here today so that Jessica and Andrew could learn more about Darcy-May. I see you've brought her Life Story Book,' she said, glancing at me. 'Thank you.' She stopped and appeared to be choosing her next words carefully.

'Before you arrived, Nia and I brought Andrew and Jessica up to date in the light of Haylea's disclosures of abuse,' she continued, her voice flat. 'They have expressed concerns about Darcy-May's health and general wellbeing. I have reassured them she is healthy and will have a medical before she goes for adoption.' This was usual practice. 'Perhaps you can reassure them too?' she said to me.

That was easy. 'Yes, Darcy-May is very healthy,' I began, addressing Andrew and Jessica. 'She's a happy, relaxed baby and is meeting all her developmental milestones. She is in a good routine and feeds every four hours, and will now go six hours at night. I'll be starting her on solid food in two months. I take her to the clinic regularly to be weighed and measured. I have brought her Red Book with me for you to see.' As I talked I dipped into my bag and placed the Red Book on the table. I didn't know what exactly they wanted to know so I hoped I was pitching it right. It was difficult to gauge, as their expressions offered no feedback. 'Darcy-May is up to date with her vaccinations,' I continued. 'She's a beautiful baby, sociable and a joy to look after. She hasn't been ill at all and doesn't have any allergies or medical conditions.'

'That you know of,' Jessica said quietly.

I stopped and looked at her questioningly.

'She might have something that you don't know about that comes out later,' she said.

'It's possible,' I replied, not really understanding.

Shari spoke. 'Jessica and Andrew are worried that if Darcy-May is the result of incest, she is more likely to have inherited genetic conditions. It may be possible to have a DNA test. It's something we're considering.'

'It's not just that,' Jessica said. 'I am horrified that the baby is a result of rape. It's sickening.'

I looked at them both and realized this was what they'd been discussing before Joy and I had arrived, which had created the tension in the room.

'It's dreadful that Haylea has been through such a shocking ordeal,' I said. 'But that won't affect Darcy-May. She's never lived at the family home. She came straight to me from the hospital.'

Andrew replied. 'That's not the issue. We were told that the biological mother was young, but we had assumed the baby was the result of a relationship.'

'That's what we all thought,' Shari said, a little defensively. 'As I explained earlier, Haylea has only just disclosed abuse.'

'I understand,' Andrew said, his face set. 'But now we know, it puts an entirely different light on our application to adopt.'

'How?' I asked.

'The baby will have the father's genes and he is a rapist,' Andrew replied bluntly.

'But Darcy-May's not going to inherit his wickedness,' I said, shocked and trying to keep my voice down. 'Babies aren't born with an evil gene. People are made and shaped by their experiences.'

'But she could inherit a tendency towards doing bad things,' Andrew said.

'There is no research evidence to suggest that is possible,' Shari pointed out.

'It's just not a nice thought,' Jessica added.

I couldn't believe we were having this conversation. I was upset and angry that they could think this way and felt very protective towards little Darcy-May. She was an innocent baby and with the right parents would grow into a healthy, well-adjusted and happy young lady. They didn't deserve her, but of course it wasn't my decision. I hoped Nia and Shari were of the same mind.

There was an awkward silence and then Joy said diplomatically to the couple: 'There is clearly a lot for you to think about. Do you have any more questions?'

'No,' Andrew said slightly brusquely. 'We need to go

away and discuss this between ourselves.' He pushed back his chair. 'Sorry to have wasted your time,' he said to me, and stood. Jessica stood too.

'I'll see you out,' Shari said, and left with them.

I was reeling from what had just taken place. It was so far from the scene I'd imagined with the happy couple poring over the photos of Darcy-May and watching the video clips I'd brought, delighted, enthralled and looking forward to meeting their daughter for the first time.

'I don't believe it!' I said to Joy and Nia, not holding back. 'What planet are they on? They've been given the chance to adopt a beautiful healthy baby that hundreds of other couples would die for. How dare they! What did they expect?' My voice caught in my throat and I blinked back tears.

Joy touched my arm reassuringly.

'Perhaps I should have given them time before the meeting to digest what I had to say,' Nia said. 'But I'm surprised by their reaction.'

'So am I,' Joy agreed.

'When you think of the conditions and disabilities that some babies are born with,' Nia said. 'And we can place them for adoption.'

'Exactly,' I said. 'I know plenty of foster carers who have worked wonders with babies who didn't have the best start in life. They come on so well with the right care. But there's nothing wrong with Darcy-May. All children come with some unknown factors, even if they're born to the parents. I have two biological children and one adopted and they all have their own personalities. Do you think they are serious about wanting to adopt?'

'I thought so,' Nia said, subdued. 'They passed all the checks and completed the adoption training.'

We were silent for a moment and then Joy said to me: 'You may as well go, Cathy. I'll speak to Shari and phone you.'

I picked up Darcy-May's Life Story Book and my bag and, saying goodbye, left the room deep in thought. I didn't see Andrew and Jessica on the way out – perhaps they'd already left or were talking to Shari in an office. I drove home incensed and affronted by their attitude. I'd known foster carers in the past who hadn't agreed with the social services' decision on where a child should live permanently, and all they could do was voice their concerns. If Jessica and Andrew still wanted to go ahead with the adoption, I would be voicing my concerns. Darcy-May, like all children, needed loving unconditionally, and I doubted they could do that.

I tried to calm down before I reached home. I'd been gone less than an hour. I was pleased to find that Haylea was no longer in her bedroom but in the living room with Ines enjoying tea and chocolate digestive biscuits. Darcy-May was lying on the sofa beside Ines, grinning and kicking her legs excitedly.

'You're back early,' Ines said.

'Yes. The meeting was cut short.'

'She's such a poppet,' Ines said, clearly besotted with Darcy-May.

'She is,' I agreed, and thought that Jessica and Andrew didn't know what they were missing.

Ines finished her tea and then I saw her out. I made Haylea and myself some lunch and then we walked to the High Street so Haylea could buy my granddaughter a card and present for her first birthday. As we walked and I pushed the buggy Haylea asked, 'Are they going to have her?'

'The couple at the adoption meeting?'

'Yes. Shari told me about them.'

It was the first time Haylea had shown any interest in Darcy-May's future, and I felt sad that I couldn't give her better news.

'I'm not sure,' I said. 'Adoption is a long process and Darcy-May deserves the best. Why do you ask?'

'I just wondered. I don't want anything bad to happen to her like it did to me.'

'It won't, love.'

CHAPTER TWENTY-TWO

NO LONGER SAFE

Emma's first birthday party on Saturday was just what I needed after Haylea's shocking disclosures and then the attitude of the couple who were supposed to be adopting Darcy-May. I was able to put all that aside and concentrate on my family and my darling granddaughter, who was now one year old. How quickly that year had passed, I thought as I drove to the party. Haylea, Paula and Darcy-May were in the car and, like me, were in the party mood.

Lucy welcomed us and it was immediately obvious the trouble she and Darren had gone to. The hall and the living room were decorated with dozens of 'Happy First Birthday' banners and balloons. On the table was a delicious cold buffet with paper party plates and napkins. Tina and Tod, Darren's parents, were already there and said they'd arrived early to help Lucy and Darren get ready. I'd met them before; they're a lovely couple and we get along very well.

The doorbell began ringing as more guests arrived – other members of Darren's family, including his sister, niece and grandparents. Adrian and Kirsty arrived, and some friends of Lucy and Darren: a couple who were also first-time parents, whom they'd got to know at ante-natal classes, and friends from work. Lucy and Darren worked at the same nursery – Lucy was on extended maternity leave and was going back part-time in January when there was a place for Emma at the nursery. I guessed there were about thirty of us and I thought of my dear mother, whose absence would be felt at all our family gatherings for many years to come. She loved family parties, as did my father. They were both children at heart.

We talked and mingled and after we'd eaten Lucy came into the living room carrying a huge birthday cake with one large sparkling candle in the middle. Emma wasn't up to blowing it out yet, but she was fascinated by it – her eyes rounded like saucers as Darren blew it out. Paula helped slice and give out the cake, then Lucy sat Emma on her lap and with Darren beside her they opened Emma's birthday presents, thanking us after each one, as we took photographs. Haylea had bought Emma a soft toy with '1 Today' on it and a nice card, which she'd signed: *All my love and best wishes, Haylea xxx*.

After the presents Haylea spent some time holding Emma's hand and walking her around the room. If anyone thought it was slightly odd that she lavished this attention on Emma while ignoring her own baby, they didn't say. I doubted many there knew of their relation-ship. To most, Darcy-May and Haylea were simply the children I was fostering.

As six o'clock approached – the time the party was due to end – Tina and I quietly began gathering together the rubbish and washing up so there wouldn't be so much to do later. It was after seven o'clock by the time we left and we hugged Lucy and Darren, saying good-bye and thanking them. It was a day to remember. Darcy-May fell asleep in the car and once home I gave her a bath and bottle, then settled her for the night. I fed her again before I went to bed and then fell asleep with happy thoughts in my head.

We had a relaxing day on Sunday. It was the beginning of August and gloriously hot. Paula, Haylea and I ate outside under the shade of the tree while Darcy-May lay on a rug. We looked at the photographs we'd taken of Emma's party and WhatsApped them to each other. I would also have some printed to frame. Later, I phoned Lucy and Darren and said what a lovely time we'd all had. They were having a relaxing day too.

On Monday Paula went to work as usual and I took Haylea in my car to see the outside of the school she would be going to in September. I didn't know if seeing it helped, but I reassured her I would take and collect her until she felt confident using the bus. On Wednesday her therapy sessions resumed and I took and collected her from that. Shari phoned later that day and made an appointment to see us the following Monday for one of her scheduled visits. She also told me that Andrew and Jessica had withdrawn their application to adopt Darcy-May and were now thinking carefully if adoption was right for them. I was relieved.

'Nia will be looking at the other applicants,' she said. 'She's sure they won't have a problem placing Darcy-May.'

'So am I. She's gorgeous.'

* * *

Although Haylea and I were aware that her father and the man who'd organized those shocking 'parties' were out on bail, and the police investigation was ongoing, she didn't want to discuss it. Since giving her interview, Haylea hadn't talked about it and seemed to be trying to forget it all, although realistically it wasn't going to be that easy. She had sleepless nights and when she did sleep she was often plagued by nightmares. I hoped therapy, time and the prosecution of her abusers would eventually help give her some closure.

The heat had been building all week and on Friday morning there was a massive thunderstorm, with lightning crackling across the sky interspersed with loud claps of thunder that made us jump. Haylea and I were in the living room watching it through the patio windows. Darcy-May was scared so I was holding her close. Sammy had bolted upstairs at the first clap of thunder and was now hiding under a bed. Haylea seemed more fascinated than scared by the storm. After a particularly loud lightning strike she said in a deadpan voice, 'It sounds like a whip cracking. I forgot to tell the police about the whips. Do you think they found them when they searched the house?'

'Whips?'

'Yes.'

'I don't know, love. You'd better tell Shari when you see her on Monday.' Part of me hoped Haylea wouldn't want to tell me any more.

'He – my father – used to crack a whip if he wanted me to do something,' she said. 'It sounded like this storm.'

'How utterly dreadful. The evil brute,' I said, holding Darcy-May even closer.

Haylea didn't say anything further and I realized she'd zoned out and gone to that far-away place that would offer some protection from the recollection. Pity I couldn't go there too, I thought, for all these shocking disclosures were playing on my mind. Although, of course, this was nothing compared to what Haylea was going through, having lived with the abuse all those years.

The storm eventually passed and the sun came out but without the oppressive heat of the last few days. After lunch I suggested to Haylea we walked to the High Street. I needed a few things, including more nappies for Darcy-May, and Haylea liked to look in the shops and spend some of her allowance. As usual I pushed Darcy-May in the buggy as Haylea walked beside me. We took a leisurely stroll to the end of the road, where we turned left onto the High Street. I bought what I needed and Haylea bought sweets and an ice cream. We retraced our footsteps towards home with Haylea still licking her ice cream, which was melting faster than she could eat it. When she'd finished I passed her a wipe so she could clean her hands and chin. 'I'm worse than a baby,' she laughed, wiping away the residue of sticky ice cream.

We entered my road and continued slowly down. It was getting hot again and I was looking forward to a cold drink. As our house came into view Haylea suddenly grabbed my arm and stopped dead.

'What is it?' I asked, following her line of vision.

'That man. No. It's OK. For a moment I thought I knew him.'

I looked and saw three people: the man Haylea had

referred to was further down the road and walking away from us; the other two were coming towards us.

'Who did you think he was?' I asked as we continued walking.

'No one,' she said. 'It's me being silly. It's happened before. I catch sight of someone and think it's one of those men coming to get me.'

By the time we reached the house the man was out of sight. I let us in, closed the front door and thought nothing more about it. Darcy-May needed her nappy changed so I took her upstairs, laid her on the bed and began to clean her. As I did I heard the front doorbell ring.

'Shall I get it?' Haylea called up.

'Yes, but check who it is in the security spyhole first.' She knew to do this anyway.

'It's a man with a parcel,' she called up.

'OK, thanks.'

I heard the front door open and then a man's voice say, 'A present from your dad.'

I ran out of my bedroom, downstairs and into the hall. The man had gone. Haylea was standing in the hall as white as a sheet and holding what looked like a shoe box. I checked outside but couldn't see anyone, and shut the front door. Before I could stop her Haylea had lifted the lid off the box. She screamed. It contained a baby doll with its head cut off. On the inside of the box lid was written in black ink: **Keep your mouth shut or else**.

Sick with fear, I tried to calm Haylea. I took the box from her and set it to one side in case it was needed for evidence. 'I'll call the police,' I said, my voice shaking. 'Do you know who he was?'

'I couldn't see his face when I looked through the spyhole, but I'm sure he's one of my father's friends,' she said, trying to catch her breath. 'He used to come to my house. I think it was him I saw in the road. They know where I am!' she cried, petrified, and grabbed my arm.

'The doors are all locked,' I said. 'So is the side gate. I'm going to fetch Darcy-May and then call the police. You go and sit in the living room.'

'No! I want to come with you,' she cried, and followed me upstairs.

Although I was trying to stay calm for Haylea's sake, I was anything but. My fingers trembled as I finished dressing Darcy-May. I knew how serious this was. I picked up the phone beside my bed and dialled 999.

'Police,' I said as the call handler asked which emergency service I wanted. Haylea was standing by me, her hand clenched into a fist and pressed to her mouth.

I was put through, gave my name and address and explained in a gabble that I was a foster carer looking after a fifteen-year-old girl who had been badly abused by her father and others, and that a man had just come to our house and threatened her. The officer had to keep stopping me to ask for clarification and more details, including Haylea's full name, her social worker's name and contact details, and when she'd first reported the abuse. She then asked to speak to Haylea, who answered more questions, beginning with if she knew the name of the man. She said Tom but didn't know his surname or where he lived. She was able to give a description of him and from what she said I learnt that he and other friends of her father had also abused her at home. There seemed to be no end to this poor girl's suffering.

Once the officer had finished speaking to Haylea, she passed the phone back to me. 'I'm going to look into this now,' she said. 'I'll get back to you.'

'What will happen?' I asked.

'If her father has broken his bail conditions, he will be rearrested and appear before the Magistrates' Court.'

'Even though it wasn't him who came to the house?'

'Yes, it's likely he's still in breach of the bail conditions, as he tried to contact Haylea through someone else. Leave it with me and I'll look into it.'

I thanked her and we said goodbye. The officer had been a lot calmer than I was, but then I supposed, given some of the issues the police have to deal with, she would have heard far worse. In the past I'd had parents come to my house when they weren't supposed to, but in all my years of fostering I'd never experienced anything as worrying as this. The paedophiles who'd been abusing Haylea and other children knew where she lived. How far would they go to silence her? The doll with a severed head was a crude but effective message. I was scared and Haylea looked petrified.

'I shouldn't have told the police,' she said.

'Yes, you should. You did right. Those men need stopping. I need to tell your social worker now.'

So with Darcy-May still lying on my bed, I telephoned Shari's mobile. It went through to voicemail and I left a message. 'It's Cathy, Haylea's carer, can you phone me, please? It's urgent. I've just had to contact the police. Haylea's father sent a man here to threaten her.'

I ended the call and tried Shari's office number. A colleague answered. 'Is Shari there? It's Cathy Glass, Haylea Walsh's foster carer.'

'She's in a meeting.'

'Can you tell her I phoned, please? It's urgent. I've left a message on her voicemail.'

'I will.'

I then telephoned Joy and she answered. I went through what had happened and said I hadn't been able to get hold of Shari as she was in a meeting. Joy appreciated the seriousness of the situation. 'Are you OK?' she thought to ask.

'Shaken, to be honest.'

'How is Haylea?'

'Very worried.'

'I'll see if I can find Shari or her manager and call you.' They worked in the same building. 'It's unlikely that man will return, but if he does, call the police.'

'I will.'

I returned the phone to its cradle and looked at Haylea. She was chewing the back of her hand. 'We've done all we can for now. Let's go downstairs.'

Her eyes filled and her bottom lip trembled. 'I'll never feel safe here again,' she said.

'Come here.' I opened my arms and she let me give her a proper hug.

I held and comforted her as best I could. 'Once your father has been rearrested, you will start to feel safe again,' I said, and prayed I was right.

Eventually Haylea began to calm down and she dried her tears. I picked up Darcy-May from where she'd been lying on the bed and we went downstairs. I settled her in the bouncing cradle and fetched her a bottle of formula. At the same time I poured Haylea and myself a glass of water each.

'What do you think is happening?' Haylea asked as I fed Darcy-May.

'I don't know. I guess someone will phone before long.'

The minutes ticked by and we continued to wait, anxious and mainly in silence. It was impossible to concentrate on anything else. At one point the letterbox on the front door suddenly snapped shut, making us both jump. I went into the hall and found an advertising flyer on the floor.

An hour passed and then my mobile rang. It was Shari. 'How is Haylea?' she asked.

'Scared.'

'I've just come off the phone to the police. They are going to rearrest her father.'

'Good.'

'But they have advised us to move Haylea straight away.'

'Oh no.'

'I'm sorry, but it's not safe for her to live with you any longer. It's not just her father and the man who came to your door who know where she is living. They are part of a larger paedophile ring. Haylea's evidence has led to further arrests, so it's likely others know she is there. We're going to move her to a hostel this evening and then find somewhere more permanent. Can you put her on, please, and I'll explain?'

'What's the matter?' Haylea asked, reading my expression.

'Shari wants to talk to you,' I said, and handed her the phone.

I sat there and watched Haylea's face crumple as Shari broke the news.

'No! I don't want to go!' she cried. 'I can stay indoors. I won't go out. Let me stay here, please. Cathy is the only family I have. I love her and she loves me.'

Tears sprang to my eyes. I moved to the sofa and sat next to Haylea as Shari continued to talk to her. Of course I didn't want her to go, but realistically I knew it was the right decision. It was the only decision they could make to protect her. But that didn't make it any easier.

Sobbing, Haylea passed the phone back to me.

'Can you pack what she needs for a few days,' Shari said to me. 'I'll arrange to have the rest of her belongings collected once she's settled.'

'Yes,' I replied numbly.

'I'll be in touch.' She said goodbye.

'Oh, Cathy, I don't want to leave,' Haylea cried, her face creasing again. 'I wish I hadn't said anything. I love you. Don't make me go.'

'It's not my decision, love,' I said, swallowing back my own tears. I put my arm around her and held her as she wept on my shoulder.

CHAPTER TWENTY-THREE

I'M SO UNHAPPY

I tried to focus on the practicalities. I knew Haylea was being moved that evening, but I didn't know by whom or when, so I thought it best to pack a bag straight away so it was ready. Once Haylea was calmer and had stopped crying, I explained I needed to put some of her things in a bag to see her through the next few days. She nodded bravely. I asked if she wanted to come and help me, but she didn't, so rather than just leave her to worry I switched on the television. Darcy-May was napping in the baby bouncer. 'Call me if she wakes,' I said, and I went up to her bedroom.

I was trying to hold it together for Haylea's sake, but inside I was falling apart. The two of us had been through so much and Haylea was supposed to be with me until she was eighteen – longer, if she wished. The poor kid. Just when she'd felt safe enough to disclose the abuse she'd suffered, her whereabouts had become known. Shari hadn't said how that had happened, but it would have been relatively easy to find her if someone had wanted to, which clearly her monster of a father had. I would keep in contact with Haylea, but once she'd gone, realistically I would no longer be on hand to give her the support and help she would need over the coming months and years.

Fighting back fresh tears, I began opening drawers, taking out her clothes and laying them on the bed. I chose those clothes that Haylea wore the most – her favourites – plus two sets of nightwear, underwear, her phone charger, shoes, coat and so on. I needed a suitcase, but they were in the loft. Then I remembered the large hold-alls she'd arrived with, which I'd put away in the storage compartment under her bed. I pulled them out and began packing. Haylea's leaving card from Waysbury and her birthday cards were still on her shelves. My eyes filled again as I carefully packed those. She had been so grate-ful for any kindness shown to her, having had none in the past. It wasn't fair she was having to leave now. Those abusers were still managing to ruin her life, even from a distance. Would she ever be free of them?

Wiping my eyes, I went into the bathroom, gathered up Haylea's toiletries and tucked them into her cosmetics bag, then I returned to her bedroom. The holdalls held a fair amount, so I was satisfied she had plenty for the first week. I zipped the bags closed and carried them down-stairs, where I put them out of sight in the front room. I returned to the living room.

The television was still on, but Haylea was staring past it into space. Darcy-May was awake and seemed to be watching Haylea.

'Do you want anything to eat?' I asked Haylea, again concentrating on the practical.

'No, thank you,' she replied, her voice sad.

I took Darcy-May from the bouncing cradle and sat with her on the floor with her toys, as I often did.

Fifteen minutes later Joy telephoned to check that Shari had called and told us what was happening. 'I am so sorry,' she said. 'You've worked wonders with Haylea. It's thanks to you she's made the progress she has.'

Her words were supposed to offer comfort, but they didn't, and I wiped a tear from the corner of my eye.

'Do you know what time Haylea is being collected?' I asked, my voice slight.

'As soon as they have found somewhere for her to go is what Shari told me. Some time this evening.' She then wound up by asking me to say goodbye to Haylea and wish her well for the future and added that she'd phone me on Monday.

'That was Joy,' I said to Haylea as I ended the call. 'She sends her best wishes.'

Haylea nodded and returned her gaze to the television.

Another half an hour passed and I was thinking I'd better make something for dinner, but then it all happened very quickly. Shari telephoned again and said the police were on their way to collect Haylea and take her to a place of safety, and asked if she was ready.

'Yes,' I replied. I thought it was a sign of just how serious this was that they were acting so quickly. 'Will I be able to see her again?' I asked.

'There is no reason why you shouldn't once she's settled, but it will be away from this area.'

She then asked to speak to Haylea and appeared to tell her what she'd told me.

'I'm going soon,' Haylea said as she handed back the phone.

'I know, love, but I will be able to see you. Did Shari tell you where you are going?'

'No, just that the police would take me and I mustn't tell anyone where it was.'

'OK. Do you need to use the bathroom? If so, go now.'

She switched off the television and went upstairs. I picked up Darcy-May, who'd had enough of lying on the floor. Haylea returned downstairs and the front doorbell rang.

'I expect that's the police,' I said. 'Wait here and I'll check.'

I took Darcy-May with me to the front door and looked through the spyhole. I could see a female police officer.

'Cathy Glass?' she asked as I opened the door.

'Yes, come in.'

'I'm here to collect Haylea Walsh.'

'We're expecting you,' I said as she stepped into the hall. I closed the front door. Haylea came out of the living room.

'All set to go?' the officer asked her.

Haylea just stared at her.

'We're rather emotional,' I said. 'Haylea was supposed to be staying with me permanently.'

'Oh dear, I am sorry.' I didn't know how much the officer knew about Haylea's circumstances or the reason for the move. 'Do you have an overnight bag?' she asked Haylea.

'There are two bags in here,' I said, and showed her into the front room.

I still had Darcy-May in my arms so couldn't help with the bags. The officer picked up one and Haylea numbly picked up the other. We went into the hall, where I took £50 from my purse and gave it to Haylea. The officer opened the front door, ready to leave. Haylea and I looked at each other.

'Take care, love,' I said, my eyes filling. 'Phone as soon as you can.'

'I will. I love you,' she said, and her tears fell.

'I love you too.'

We only hugged briefly. The officer was already out the door and I knew that prolonging our goodbye would only make it worse. 'You'd better go,' I said.

Haylea nodded and followed the officer down the front path as I stood at the door holding Darcy-May. I watched Haylea get into the back of the police car as the officer put her bags in the boot. It was a lovely summer evening, a cruel contrast to our forced separation. Haylea looked at me through her side window, but it was that blank, far-away gaze that meant the present was too painful to bear. I waved as the car pulled away, but she didn't respond. I went indoors, closed the front door and, with Darcy-May in my arms, I cried openly. That poor girl.

It was some time before I felt like doing anything. I sat on the sofa holding Darcy-May and worried about Haylea. Then Darcy-May began to grizzle for a bottle so I gave her the rest of the one she'd started earlier. I realized Paula would be home soon from work so after I'd fed Darcy-May I took her into the kitchen and tried to think what I could make for dinner. I wasn't hungry — my stomach was knotted in a tight ball — but Paula would need something. I opened the freezer door, saw a lasagne I'd previously made and, with no enthusiasm, I took it out and put it in the oven. I should tell Paula, Adrian and Lucy that Haylea had gone. I decided to text them now and then phone when I could tell them without bursting into tears.

I went into the living room, sat on the sofa with Darcy-May beside me and sent a message to our WhatsApp group: *I'm very sorry but Haylea has had to leave us. She's just been moved by the police to a safe house. I'll explain later. Love you, Mum x*

OMG! What happened? Lucy messaged back straight away with an emoji of a shocked face.

I'll phone you tonight x, I replied.

Are you OK? Adrian texted.

Yes. Speak soon x. I knew he'd be on his way home from work.

Paula phoned from the bus and I told her what had happened, pausing every so often to fight back fresh tears. Of course she was as shocked and upset as I was, but said stoically, 'I suppose if she was in danger they had to move her.'

'Yes. There was no choice. Paula, I'm sure that man won't come back here, and her father has been rearrested, but just be aware.'

'I will. They're horrible people.'

'Evil bastards.'

'Mum, you don't normally swear.'

'I know. Take care. I'll see you soon.'

I missed Haylea already and knew she'd be missing me. She'd never had a proper mother and I'd been more than happy to fulfil that role. Since she'd come to live with us she'd hardly left my side. Even when she wasn't in the same room I could hear her elsewhere in the house. She'd fitted easily into my family and had been so grateful for everything I'd done for her. My eyes watered again. She'd had a new life ahead of her. A new school – we were going to buy her uniform the following week – where she was hoping to make new friends. All that had been taken away from her by her bloody father and those other evil bastards. Hadn't they caused her enough pain? Why couldn't they just leave her alone? But of course I knew why. Haylea's evidence was going to help convict them. I hoped it still would and they were all sent to prison for a very long time.

I heard Paula's key go in the front door and I went into the hall. We gave each other a very big hug. Sometimes a hug can say more than a thousand words.

'Haylea was such a nice person,' Paula said. 'It's not fair.'

'I know.'

'Have you heard anything from her?'

'No, not yet.'

Paula went upstairs to have a wash and change out of her office clothes, then we had dinner. There was a big gap at the table where Haylea should have been. Darcy-May, in the bouncing cradle, seemed to think so too. She appeared to be frowning as she looked at the empty chair. Paula agreed.

'Was Haylea upset at leaving Darcy-May?' she asked.

'No, just us.' Paula appreciated why.

'Where do you think they've taken her?'

'I don't know. Shari said she was going to a hostel out of the area tonight and then they'd find her somewhere more permanent. I hope it's with another foster carer. She didn't do well in the children's home.'

We finished our dinner, subdued and speculating about Haylea. Thankfully Paula had already made arrangements to go to the cinema with a friend that evening, otherwise I think we would have been very poor company for each other. She left soon after dinner and I saw her off at the door.

'Take care,' I called after her.

It was still light outside, but it crossed my mind that now Paula had a permanent job she could afford to run a car. She'd passed her test a while ago and had been thinking about buying a car. It would be safer than using the bus, especially late at night.

After Paula had gone I spent time with Darcy-May and then began her bath and bedtime routine slightly earlier than usual so I could phone Lucy and Adrian as I'd promised.

Needless to say, they were both shocked and saddened to hear the circumstances in which Haylea had left. Although Adrian hadn't wanted me to foster an older child after he'd moved out, he'd never criticized my decision to take Haylea. Indeed, he and Kirsty had welcomed Haylea unreservedly, although they'd never known the details of her past. There was no need. Adrian has always been sensitive and often internalizes his feelings.

'I am so sorry, Mum. You did your best,' was all he said.

While Lucy – far more expressive and feisty – exclaimed down the phone, 'I hate those effing men. They need castrating.'

I couldn't disagree.

Lucy continued to lambast Haylea's abusers and others like them who preyed on children and ruined lives. So many of the children we'd fostered had been sexually abused. It seemed to be endemic.

'I'll let you know as soon as I hear anything more about Haylea,' I said, winding up.

'Thanks. And Mum –'

'Yes?'

'Guess who sent Emma a late birthday card?'

'Bonnie?'

'It arrived today. She's written in the card that she will see us before long.'

'OK. Good.'

Bonnie was Lucy's birth mother and they saw each other once or twice a year at the most, when it suited Bonnie. She had last visited Lucy unexpectedly when Emma had been ten days old and it hadn't gone well. I'd telephoned Bonnie afterwards and smoothed things over but Lucy hadn't seen her since. She had grown to accept her birth mother's shortcomings, as I had, and while she was happy to see her every so often, she didn't want any more. Neither did Bonnie, who, although not a bad person, continued to face many struggles in her own life. Lucy preferred to meet her at a coffee shop rather than at home.

'I'm going to make it on a day when Darren can come too,' Lucy added.

'Yes. All right, love.'

Then, promising Lucy again I'd let her know when I had any more news about Haylea, I said goodbye.

It was nearly 10 p.m. and I was exhausted. I decided I wouldn't wait up for Paula. Although Darcy-May usually slept for a six-hour stretch at night – not bad for a five-month-old baby – it couldn't be guaranteed, and six hours wasn't really enough for me. The lack of sleep plus the trauma of recent days had finally caught up with me and I could have fallen asleep on the sofa.

Shattered, I hauled myself out of the chair. Sammy, aware it was his bedtime too, stretched, ready to follow me into the kitchen-diner where he spent the night. My mobile rang. Too late for a friend to be calling for a chat, I thought as I picked up the phone. Haylea's name was on the display. Relief flooded through me until I heard her voice.

'Oh Cathy, I'm so unhappy. I don't want to live any more.'

CHAPTER TWENTY-FOUR

DISTRESSING CALLS

'Haylea, where are you?' I asked.

'I don't know,' she sobbed. 'Miles away in a hostel.'

'Is someone there with you?'

'No. I'm alone in a tiny room.'

'A room in the hostel?'

'Yes. They give the bigger rooms to the women with children.' So I assumed she was in a women's refuge. 'I want to come home and be with you.'

'Oh, love. I wish you could have stayed, but it wasn't safe.'

'I don't care. I'd rather be dead than here.'

'Don't say that, please. It's late and you've had a very traumatic day. Try to get some sleep and you'll feel better in the morning.'

'No, I won't,' she sobbed. 'I don't want to live any more.'

I was very worried and, being so far away, there was little I could do to help.

'Is there someone there – a member of staff – you can talk to?'

'I don't know. I guess so. Some of the staff sleep here. All the other women are older than me and most of them have kids.'

'It's a women's refuge.'

'It was the only place that could take me tonight. I was in the police car for ages. We didn't arrive until nine o'clock.'

'It's only temporary,' I said. 'Shari said they will find you something more suitable.'

'But not until next week!' Haylea cried.

'Is that what Shari said?'

'Yes. She phoned while I was in the police car. It's because it's the weekend.'

'I know it's not ideal, but you're safe there. No one knows where you are.' I knew something of women's refuges from having done some voluntary work in one some years before. They were occasionally used for teenage girls fleeing danger, but it was difficult to know what to say to Haylea to make her feel better.

'Can you get into bed and listen to your music like you used to here?' I tried.

'Is Paula there?' she asked.

'She's at the cinema with a friend. Lucy, Adrian and Paula send their love. They are sorry you've had to leave but understand why.'

'Will I see you all again?' Haylea asked, her voice breaking. It was pitiful and I was struggling to hold back my tears.

'Shari said once you're settled.'

'I hate my life.'

I was choked up and even more angry with her father. Haylea had been making progress and would have continued to do so had it not been for him.

'Haylea, I know you're feeling low at the moment, but think how far you've come. You're been so brave in the past and I know you can be brave again. This is another hurdle to overcome. You can do it. Don't let him get the better of you.'

I heard what sounded like a knock on a door, and Haylea said a tentative, 'Yes?'

'Can I come in?' a woman asked.

'Yes,' Haylea replied.

I heard the door open and then the woman say, 'I'm making a cup of tea. Would you like one?'

Haylea sniffed and I could picture her wiping away her tears as she used to here.

'You're upset,' the woman said kindly. 'Come down when you've finished on the phone and we can talk.'

'OK,' Haylea said, and I heard the door close.

'Was that one of the staff?' I asked.

'Yes.'

'Go down and have a cup of tea with her and we'll talk again tomorrow.'

'I will,' Haylea said quietly, and we ended the call.

Thank goodness she had some company, I thought. I couldn't bear the idea of her being upset and alone in a strange room. I continued with my night-time routine: saw Sammy into his bed, poured myself a glass of water, then closed the door to the kitchen-diner and went upstairs to bed.

Darcy-May would wake for a feed around midnight and I was hoping to get an hour's sleep before then. However, I was still awake at 11 p.m. worrying about Haylea. I heard Paula quietly let herself in and go to bed. Half an hour later my phone began vibrating from where I'd left it on the bed. Usually I switched it off at night unless I was on standby for an emergency foster placement, but that wasn't so tonight. I'd left my phone on in case Haylea called, as I wanted to be there for her. It was her and I answered it quietly so I wouldn't wake Darcy-May.

'I can't sleep,' Haylea said. 'It's all going through my head. All those horrible things they made me do. I can't shut them out. I started to tell my therapist last week.'

She wasn't crying but sounded very low.

'You can talk to me,' I said. 'And the staff there.'

'No, I can't, it's too awful. I can't tell you.' Then, changing the subject, she asked, 'Do you think Shari could find my brothers and sister?' I knew that Haylea had two older brothers, one of whom was in prison. Her sister, also older, had run way from home shortly after their mother had left. That was all I knew about them. Haylea had never mentioned them before and I could understand why she had now – alone in a strange room, miles from anywhere, they were the only family she had. Normally the social services kept siblings in contact if there was a bond, but I didn't know if Shari knew how to trace them or if, indeed, it was in Haylea's best interests to do so.

'You will need to talk to Shari about that,' I said.

'I can hear a baby crying,' Haylea said, changing the subject again.

'Did someone explain to you what a women's refuge is?'

'Yes, the police lady. She told me it was for women escaping violent partners, so I mustn't tell anyone where it was. She said their lives could be in danger if they found out where they were.'

'That's true.'

'Was my life in danger?'

'It certainly wasn't safe for you to stay here.'

We continued talking, Haylea going from one subject to another. I kept my voice low, but Darcy-May began to wake for a feed.

'I'll have to go,' I said. 'Darcy-May needs a bottle. Try to get some sleep and phone me tomorrow if you want to.'

We said goodnight. I went downstairs, warmed a bottle of formula and returned to my bedroom to feed Darcy-May. Once she was settled again in her cot, I got back into bed and finally fell asleep, my phone on silent beside me. Haylea didn't call again that night so I assumed she must have slept too. I didn't hear from her again until four o'clock the following afternoon and she sounded brighter. 'I've made a friend,' she said.

'Excellent.'

'Tammy is nineteen and has two children. The kid's father has been beating her up. She didn't have time to pack before she left. He was going to kill her. She has been here for three months and is waiting for council accommodation.'

While it was another sad story, I was pleased Haylea had someone she could call a friend. However, that night, when she was alone in her room again, the horror of her past came back to haunt her. At 2 a.m. I was woken by my phone vibrating. 'Haylea, just a minute,' I said quietly. 'I don't want to wake Darcy-May.'

I got out of bed and went quietly round the landing to Haylea's old bedroom, where I closed the door so I wouldn't wake Darcy-May or Paula.

'I'm sorry to disturb you,' she said. 'But I had another nightmare. He was here in my room. It seemed so real. I've got the light on.'

I assumed *he* was her father.

I talked to Haylea, reassuring her for over an hour until she felt able to try to go to sleep. I didn't say anything significant, nothing I hadn't said before, but I think just having someone on the end of the phone helped – she didn't feel so alone.

The following day, Sunday, I didn't hear from Haylea and I allowed myself to hope she was feeling a bit better. But that night her terror returned and we were on the phone for two hours, between midnight and two o'clock. Again, I took the call in her old room. I had stayed up to give Darcy-May a bottle, so I hadn't had any sleep yet. It was nearly 3 a.m. before I was able to fall asleep, then Darcy-May woke at 5.45 for a feed. I went back to bed and didn't hear Paula get up and go to work. When I woke it was nearly 9 a.m. I checked my phone and found a text from Paula: *I hope I didn't wake you. Have a good day. Love P xx.*

Thanks, love xx, I replied.

I showered, dressed and got Darcy-May up, all the time thinking of Haylea and wondering how she was getting on. Just because a looked-after child is no longer with a foster carer doesn't mean we stop worrying about them. Indeed, we often worry more until we are reassured they are happy and doing well.

Joy telephoned that Monday morning to ask how Haylea's move had gone. I told her, including Haylea's distressing night-time phone calls. She said she'd try to speak to Shari to find out when she would be moved from the hostel. I had emailed Shari. I was also updating my log notes on Haylea. I thought it wise to keep those going until Haylea was with a permanent foster carer who would be keeping records of their own.

Haylea's next call came that evening, and although not distressed, she sounded down. She said there was nothing for her to do as all the other women in the hostel spent most of their time with their children. She hadn't seen Tammy as her youngest child was ill, so she'd stayed in her room. Haylea asked to speak to Paula and I heard Paula asking her questions and trying to cheer her up.

'She really isn't happy there,' Paula said when they'd finished.

'I know, love. Hopefully Shari will find her somewhere else soon.'

It was a worry and there was nothing we could do. I didn't even know where Haylea was.

She phoned again that night. I was half expecting her call. While she'd been with me she hadn't slept well but had usually stayed in bed and listened to music. Now it seemed that at night her dark thoughts were getting the better of her as the horrors of her past closed in. Again, I took the call in Haylea's old bedroom. She didn't really have much to say, beyond that she was fed up with everything and missed us dreadfully. She asked what we'd been doing and again I tried to reassure her that things would get better. After an hour or so I said I needed to go to bed to get a few hours' sleep before Darcy-May woke, and reluctantly we said goodbye.

Shari didn't phone until Wednesday, but thankfully she had some good news.

'We've found Haylea a foster placement. We're moving her tomorrow – Thursday. They are a married couple, husband and wife, experienced foster carers, who have two teenagers there already – one is their own son and the other a looked-after child.'

'Excellent,' I said.

'Will it be all right if I give the carers your phone number so you can tell them a bit about Haylea and her routine.'

'Yes, of course.' It was usual to pass this sort of information on either by phone or email. 'Does Haylea know yet?'

'Yes, I've just told her. The other piece of good news is that Family Finding have identified an excellent match for Darcy-May.'

'OK,' I said less enthusiastically.

'A childless couple in their early thirties. They are already approved to adopt. Nia is going to set up a meeting for us all. She'll be in touch to arrange it. Take your photographs and Life Story Book.'

'And they are aware of the circumstances of Darcy-May's birth?' I checked.

'Yes, Nia has told them as much as we know.'

Was I reassured? Only partly. We'd already had one 'excellent match' go nowhere. I didn't doubt the integrity of these childless couples who wanted to adopt, but I felt that sometimes their enthusiasm for wanting a family got in the way of reality. I knew of adoptions that had failed or struggled (see my books *Nobody's Son* and *A Long Way from Home*), sometimes within a very short time. Others failed years later, often when the child hit puberty and started to challenge their parents and test their love and commitment for them. If parents gave up on the young person, they were left bruised, battered and feeling unlovable. I'm sure the parents suffered too, as it's never an easy decision, so it was important to get it right.

Once Shari had finished, I texted Haylea.

Good luck with the move tomorrow xx.

I purposely wasn't phoning Haylea as her bond with me needed to gradually loosen so she could transfer her attachment to her permanent long-term carer. Or that's the thinking in fostering, anyway.

Five minutes later Haylea phoned.

'I'm pleased to be leaving the hostel,' she said. 'But I wish I could come and live with you again.'

I felt awful. 'I know, love, so do I, but you understand why it's not possible.'

'I guess. Shari said the carers have other young people there my age, so I'll have company.'

'Good. It might be a bit strange to begin with so give yourself time. How is Tammy's child?' I thought to ask.

'Better. We're going to the park later.'

'That'll be nice.'

'I like the parks near you better.'

'I'm sure there will be other nice parks near where your new carers live,' I said positively. 'Are you seeing them before you move in?' It was usual before a planned move.

'No, they're busy. They are going to phone me later.'

'They are phoning me too. I'll let them know what you like to do in your spare time – baking, days out. What else?'

'Helping you.'

'I'm sure they'll appreciate that.'

'I'd rather help you.'

Every comment I made Haylea turned around by saying how much she missed us and wanted to return. I felt I was doing her more harm than good. Then I heard Darcy-May wake from her nap. 'I'll have to go now, love. Darcy-May is awake. Good luck for tomorrow. I'll be thinking of you.'

'I'll be thinking of you too,' Haylea said, her voice catching.

We said goodbye.

It was very sad, but I knew from years of fostering that once Haylea was settled with her new family she should start to feel better. I would feel happier too once I'd spoken to the new carers and been able to tell them of Haylea's needs and how best to meet them. I was expecting them to call that day, but it was the following morning before they phoned, and, far from feeling reassured, I had concerns.

CHAPTER TWENTY-FIVE

MISSING

Haylea didn't phone me during the night, although that didn't stop me from waking every so often to check my phone.

At ten o'clock in the morning her new foster carer called. I had Darcy-May in one hand and a bottle of formula in the other.

'Cathy, its Celia Marchant,' she said in a loud, confident voice. 'I'm going to be Haylea's new foster carer.'

'Thanks for calling,' I said, sitting on the sofa with the phone lodged under my chin so I could feed Darcy-May.

'Shari asked me to call you, but I've spoken to Haylea and I don't anticipate any problems,' she said. 'Shari has sent the Essential Information Forms and we're used to fostering teenagers. That's the only age they send us now.' She gave a low, cynical laugh.

'How was Haylea when you spoke to her?' I asked.

'She didn't say much, which makes a change from some of those we've had.'

'Haylea isn't really like other teenagers,' I said. 'She doesn't have much confidence and can be very introverted and withdrawn. She wants to please and be liked.'

'That'll be a first here!' Celia quipped with another laugh.

'She needs a lot of reassurance and can easily become frightened. She has nightmares about her past. Are you aware of what happened to her?'

'She's been sexually abused and there is a court case pending,' Celia said, which hardly did justice to what Haylea had been through.

I explained in more detail so Celia was better equipped to give Haylea the help she needed. While I was talking, she said 'of course' a few times as though I was telling her what she already knew, but each child's needs are different. I then began going through Haylea's routine, including, 'She likes a long bath in the morning, but I've told her she'll have to have it in the evening once she's at school.'

'It's a shower here,' Celia said brusquely. 'The kids are given half an hour each evening. We have a rota. My husband and I have our own en-suite.'

'OK,' I said, acknowledging that carers did things differently. 'Haylea's got some of her belongings with her, but the rest of her things are still with me as she was moved at short notice.'

'Sorry, Cathy, I am going to have to stop you there,' Celia said. 'We're due to collect Haylea in fifteen minutes. Don't worry yourself. She'll be fine. She's going to have to be – we're the only carers for miles willing to take a teenager. I'll get her to call you once she's settled.'

'Thank you,' I said, and the call was ended.

* * *

I put Darcy-May's empty bottle on the coffee table and lightly rubbed her back to release any trapped wind. As I did, I gave myself a telling off. You're not the only one who knows how to look after Haylea. Just because Celia's approach is different from yours doesn't mean it's wrong and she won't meet Haylea's needs. Foster carers are very different people, individuals; there is no mould, you know that. Give the poor woman a chance. She's an experienced foster carer like you. Haylea will be fine.

As the day passed I thought about Haylea meeting her new carers for the first time and then being taken home – wherever that was. I hoped she got on with the other young people in the house – they were a similar age to her – and it would be good for her to have a caring, reliable father figure.

I took Darcy-May to the clinic that afternoon to be weighed and checked over, and by the time I was preparing dinner I was less worried about Haylea. Now she was at her new home and had met her family she should be feeling relieved, if not happier. Celia had said she would remind Haylea to phone me once she had settled in, but I wasn't expecting her call for a week or even longer. When a child leaves a foster carer to go to permanency it's usual to wait a few weeks before phoning or seeing the child, otherwise it's thought it could be unsettling for them.

Paula arrived home from work and asked straight away if I'd heard anything from Haylea.

'It's a bit soon yet, but I'm sure the move went well,' I said positively.

* * *

That night, purely out of habit, I left my mobile phone on. I wasn't expecting Haylea to call. She'd been lonely at the hostel and anxious after having to suddenly leave us. Now she was with her permanent foster carers she'd feel safe. I fed Darcy-May just before midnight and then got into bed. Before I'd fallen asleep my mobile began vibrating on the bedside cabinet. I quickly picked it up and saw Haylea's name on the display. 'Just a minute,' I said in a whisper, getting out of bed. 'I don't want to wake Darcy-May.' I went round the landing and into Haylea's old bedroom. 'Hello, love, it's very late. How are you?'

'I'm so unhappy. I hate it here,' she said, her voice catching. 'I want to come home to you.'

That wasn't possible and I knew I had to be reasonably firm. 'Haylea, you've only just arrived, love. I told you it could seem strange at first. You need to give yourself time. You know you can't live with me. It's not safe.'

'I hate my life. I wish I was dead.'

'No, you don't. You've been through far more than a change in foster carer in the past. You can do this, Haylea. I know you can.'

'I don't want to stay here.'

'You've got to give it a chance, love. Have you met everyone there? What have you been doing?' I asked, hoping to get her talking about something positive.

'Nothing. I unpacked and then stayed in my room.'

'What, the whole time?'

'Yes.'

'Have you spoken to the other young people there?'

'Not really. There are two fifteen-year-old boys – one's the carers' son and the other is in foster care. Celia said they might be having another girl next week.'

'Did you all haver dinner together?'

'No, they wanted me to, but I stayed in my room, so Celia brought it up on a tray.'

'Well, tomorrow I think you should try to go down and join them.'

'I'll try,' Haylea said, then lowered her voice and added, 'I don't really like them.'

'You have to give it a chance,' I said again.

We talked for a few minutes longer – with me trying to be positive and lift Haylea's mood – but all she wanted to do was reflect on her time with me and how much she was missing us.

Suddenly she broke off mid-sentence. 'Sshh, I can hear someone coming.'

A second later I heard Celia say, 'Haylea, I'm coming in.' Then she said, 'I allowed you to keep your phone with you tonight so you could listen to music to help you sleep, not to chat.'

Oh shit, I thought.

'Who are you talking to?' Celia asked. 'It's after midnight.'

'Cathy,' Haylea replied, subdued.

'Put Celia on and I'll explain,' I said.

Celia came on the phone. 'Hello, Cathy.' I could tell by her tone that she was annoyed with me, and who could blame her?

'I am sorry,' I said. 'Haylea couldn't sleep and phoned me as she used to do at the hostel. I hope she didn't wake you.'

'No, I was just coming up to bed. We don't allow phones, iPads or other devices in the bedrooms at night, but we made an exception for Haylea as it was her first night and she said listening to music helped her sleep.'

'I fully understand,' I said. 'I have the same rules here, but Haylea got used to phoning me at night if she needed to talk.'

'She knows she can talk to me,' Celia said rather curtly. 'If she phones you again, I'd be grateful if you didn't answer or she will never settle here. Now, it's very late and she needs to get some sleep.'

'Yes, of course. Can I just say goodnight?'

She returned the phone to Haylea. 'Night, love,' I said. 'Try to go to sleep. You'll feel better in the morning.'

'Night, Cathy,' Haylea said in a small voice that broke my heart. 'Sorry I got you into trouble.'

'Don't worry, but it's probably better if you don't phone me again at night.'

I felt dreadful saying it, but Celia's request was reasonable.

'Night, love,' I said again, and ended the call.

I returned to my bedroom and thought about Haylea until I fell asleep.

Haylea didn't call or text again that night or the next, which I hoped was a good sign, although I thought about her often and worried. On Saturday Paula was up earlier than I would have expected for the weekend. 'Adrian is picking me up at ten o'clock,' she said. 'We're going to look at some cars.'

'Wonderful. How exciting.'

We'd had a chat about her buying a car and Adrian knew a fair amount about cars, having owned an old one that he'd repaired himself before he'd been able to afford a newer model.

'I'll give you something towards the cost of it,' I offered.

'Thanks, Mum.'

However, I always treated my children equally, so whatever I gave to Paula I would give to Lucy and Adrian to do with as they wished.

When Adrian arrived to collect Paula he came in for a coffee and a chat. Kirsty wasn't with him as she was seeing a friend. Once he and Paula had left, I took Darcy-May to the High Street. I only needed a few groceries so it shouldn't have taken long, but I kept stopping and talking to people I knew. Having lived in the same area for nearly thirty years, I knew a lot of people, and I do like a chat. It was a fine day and on my way home I sat in the park to give Darcy-May her bottle, where I got chatting to an elderly neighbour.

It was nearly four o'clock when Adrian dropped off Paula, and they'd had success. One garage they'd been to had a car that ticked all the boxes, but it was at one of their other branches, some miles away. They were arranging to have the car brought to their local showroom for the following Saturday, when Paula could take it for a test drive. She was very excited, as was I. Becoming a car owner is a milestone.

That night I didn't switch off my phone as Celia had asked, and thankfully Haylea didn't phone me. Would I have answered if she had? Probably, but I would have kept the conversation short. Having heard first-hand from Haylea the horrors of her suffering and seen how terrified she could become at night, I wouldn't refuse to speak to her if she was in distress. Hopefully in time she would transfer her attachment to Celia and be able to confide in her.

I didn't hear anything from Haylea on Sunday either so by Monday I was allowing myself to believe that no news was good news.

That was until the police arrived.

It was three o'clock on Monday afternoon and I answered the front door with Darcy-May in my arms to find two uniformed officers standing there. 'Cathy Glass?'

'Yes,' I said, going cold. I immediately assumed the worst and that one of my family had been involved in a road traffic accent. 'What's happened?'

'There is nothing for you to worry about, but we understand you used to foster Haylea Walsh,' the lead officer said.

'Yes, I did,' I replied, and felt another stab of fear.

'Haylea has been reported missing by her foster carer and she thought she might be here.'

A mixture of relief and concern flooded through me. 'No, she's not. Why didn't Celia phone me? I could have told her.'

'It's usual in a missing persons investigation to visit the places where they might be,' the lead officer said. Which I knew from my own experience of having to report looked-after children missing. 'Can we come in and have a look around.'

'Yes. Of course.' Again, this was normal procedure. 'When did she go missing?' I asked, worried.

'Very early this morning before the carers were up. She's taken her phone and some money, but no clothes. Has she been in touch with you?'

'Not since Thursday night,' I said. 'She phoned me around midnight feeling very low. Have you spoken to her social worker?' I asked.

'Yes. As a result of what she told us Haylea has been classified as a high-risk missing person. Her details have been circulated and we're actively looking for her.' I assumed she'd been categorized as high risk because of her fragile mental state; that she was a looked-after child and had previously tried to commit suicide. It was very worrying.

We went into the living room and I told the officers about the last conversation I'd had with Haylea. Shari had explained her background. Then I stayed in the living room with Darcy-May on my lap as the officers went from room to room, including upstairs. Satisfied Haylea wasn't there, they returned downstairs.

'Do you have any idea where she might have gone?' the lead officer asked.

'None at all,' I said. I'd been thinking about it. 'She doesn't have any real friends and she certainly wouldn't go home or to Waysbury Children's Home. That's where she was before she came to me. Can't you track her phone?' I asked.

'It's been switched off all day. Her carers thought she might have called you.'

'No, not since Thursday.'

'If she does, please contact us straight away.' The lead officer handed me a business card. 'And tell Haylea to either go to her foster carers' or to a place of safety and tell someone,' he added.

'I will.'

I saw the officers out and then anxiously racked my brain, trying to think where Haylea might have gone. Could she be making her way back to me? I didn't know how far away the foster carers lived, but from what

Haylea and Shari had said it was a long way. Perhaps she was using buses and trains to try to find her way back. It was the best scenario I could imagine, for the alternative – that she was so depressed she was suicidal – was too awful to contemplate.

I thought back to our last conversation on Thursday night and wondered if I could have done more. Could I have said something that would have helped her? Or, heaven forbid, had I inadvertently said something that had made it worse? Sometimes as a parent or foster carer you really struggle to get it right and know what to say for the best.

I tried calling Haylea's mobile, but as the officers had said it was switched off. I tried again fifteen minutes later with the same result. I was worried sick and praying for her return. Haylea wasn't streetwise. She was a vulnerable young woman who could easily be taken advantage of.

I tried her phone again and then every fifteen minutes or so, willing her to answer or at least switch it on. When Paula arrived home from work at six o'clock she knew straight away from my expression that something was wrong.

'Haylea is missing,' I said. 'She disappeared early this morning before her carers were up and no one has heard from her since.'

Paula appreciated the seriousness of the situation and was equally worried. She offered to take Darcy-May upstairs with her while she got changed, while I put together some dinner. We ate talking about Haylea and speculating where she might be.

I continued to try Haylea's phone throughout the

evening. I also phoned Celia to check Haylea hadn't been found and no one had thought to tell me.

'No, we haven't heard from her,' Celia said, a little tartly.

'If you hear anything can you let me know, please?'

'Yes, of course.'

I kept trying Haylea's phone and then just before 10 p.m. my mobile rang. It was her. Relief flooded through me, but it was short-lived.

'Cathy,' she said in a tiny, shaky voice. 'Thank you for being so kind to me. I just wanted to say goodbye.' And she ended the call.

CHAPTER TWENTY-SIX

KELLIE

With my heart racing I called Haylea straight back, but she didn't answer. Her phone was still on and I let the call ring out. I tried again, but it just kept ringing. She had sounded desperate and the finality of that good-bye made my blood run cold.

I tried her phone again and then I texted.

Haylea, love, answer your phone, please. Nothing is so bad we can't put it right xx.

Ten minutes later I phoned again, but she didn't answer, then a text arrived.

Are you angry with me?

No, of course not. I am very worried about you. I'll phone now. Please answer. We will work out what to do for the best xx.

I gave her a few seconds to read the text and then phoned. Mercifully she answered my call.

'Well done, love,' I said.

'Oh Cathy, I'm so unhappy. I don't want to live any more. I hate it here. I hate my life. No one cares.'

'Haylea, a lot of people care and are worried about you. The police came here earlier looking for you. Where are you now?'

'At the back of a pub.'

'Where?'

'I don't know. After I left Celia's I went to a shopping centre, but it closed at eight o'clock so I came here. It's busy with lots of people in the garden. No one is bothering with me.'

'But you can't stay there, love. We need to sort this out. Tell me what I can do to help. You were getting on well when you were here.'

'I don't know what you can do,' she said with a small sob. 'It's all so horrible. I hate my life and I don't like Celia and her family.'

'You haven't really been there very long,' I said gently.

'Long enough,' she replied, and, despite everything, I had to smile.

'Oh Haylea. What can I do? Would it help if I spoke to Shari tomorrow and asked her if she could find you somewhere different to live? I'm not promising she will agree, but would it help?' I was aware that sometimes placements didn't work out for any number of reasons.

'I guess, but where would I go? I didn't like that children's home. Only Cook was nice to me there.'

'Shari will have to try to find a better match for you,' I said. 'If I promise to speak to her, will you go back to Celia's for tonight?'

'She'll be angry with me and I don't know how to get there.'

'She won't be angry. She'll be relieved you have been found. I could call her and ask her or her husband to come to collect you.'

'All right, but just for tonight, then you'll speak to Shari tomorrow?'

'Yes, I will. Now, we need to work out where you are. What's the name of the pub?'

'I don't know.'

'There should be a sign somewhere with the name of it. Maybe at the front? Can you look while I stay on the phone?'

It went quiet and then I heard talking and laughing in the background. It was a warm summer evening and Haylea had said the pub garden was busy.

'The sign says "The Royal Oak",' Haylea said at last.

'Good. Can you wait somewhere safe out the front while I call Celia?'

She went quiet and then said, 'You know you said the police were looking for me, well, there's a police car just pulled up outside the pub. Do you think they are looking for me?'

'Maybe, but even if they're not, you are registered as missing on the police computer. I want you to go to them now – I'll stay on the phone. Tell them who you are and you've been reported missing.'

'They won't be angry with me, will they?' Haylea asked.

'No, love. They will be relieved too.'

'Will they know where Celia lives?'

'Yes.'

I stayed on the phone and a minute later I heard Haylea say, 'Excuse me, my name is Haylea Walsh and my foster carer has reported me missing.'

I couldn't hear the officer's reply, but I breathed a huge sigh of relief. Whether the police had traced her phone now it was turned on or it was pure chance they'd turned up I didn't know, but she was safe. I stayed on the phone and could hear a conversation between the officers and Haylea, before she said to me: 'They are going to take me to Celia's.'

'I'll phone Shari in the morning. Goodnight, love.'

'Goodnight.'

Of course I went straight upstairs to Paula and told her Haylea had been found. She too was relieved and delighted.

'Thank goodness she phoned you,' Paula said.

'Yes, indeed.'

I was still on a high from all the drama of the evening, so I waited up to give Darcy-May a late feed. Just as I was getting into bed Haylea texted.

I'm back. Don't forget to phone Shari xx.

I won't xx, I replied.

At 9 a.m. the following morning I telephoned Shari. She'd just arrived in the office and was checking emails.

'You know Haylea was found late last night,' I began.

'Yes, I'm just reading the report now. She was found at ten-thirty outside a public house in –' She named the area.

'Yes, I don't know if your report includes her reasons for running away, but she told me it was because she was desperately unhappy at Celia's. I promised her I'd phone you to see if she could move to another carer.'

'I see,' Shari said, slightly wearily. I guessed she really didn't need this on top of an already huge workload. 'I'll speak to Haylea and her carer now.'

'I've made it clear to Haylea that she can't come back here,' I emphasized. 'I think she accepts that, but she is unhappy there.'

'I understand,' Shari said, and wound up the call.

I texted Haylea: *I've phoned Shari and she will be in touch with you.*

I didn't hear any more until 4 p.m. when Shari phoned.

'I've spoken to Haylea and her foster carer. There are no carers free in the county where Haylea is now, but there is one in the neighbouring county. She's a new carer with no experience of looking after teenagers. She is a single parent with a seven-year-old daughter. I've spoken to her and she's worried she isn't up to looking after Haylea, but she's agreed to take her for a few days until somewhere more suitable can be found.'

'All right,' I said tentatively.

'I've explained this to Haylea and she wants to go there, although she knows it will mean another move. The carer has asked to speak to you, so I'll give her your number.'

'Yes, fine.'

We said goodbye.

Although Haylea had wanted to go to the new carer short term, rather than stay where she was, it meant that when she made the next move she would have had four foster carers in little over a week. Not ideal, but I've heard of worse. Some care-leavers who have contacted me have had upwards of fifty moves during their time in care. Some were unavoidable, but others could have been avoided if the carers had been better matched with the child or more support had been put in.

An hour later Kellie, Haylea's new foster carer, telephoned.

'I'm brand new to all of this,' she said, with a small, nervous laugh. 'I was only approved to foster yesterday.'

'Well done,' I said, congratulating her. She was softly spoken with a slight north-country accent.

'I know I'm only having Haylea for a few days because there is no one else, but I am worried,' she said. 'Haylea has been through so much, I don't want to get it wrong and make it worse.'

I immediately warmed to her. She seemed open to advice. I proceeded to tell her all about Haylea, including her past, her disclosures, the police investigation, her routine, needs, likes, dislikes and how she could zone out if she couldn't cope with something. 'I'm not sure if hearing all this helps you or makes it worse,' I ended.

'I'm not sure either,' she said with the same nervous laugh. 'Can I phone you if I've got any questions?'

'Yes, of course. What time are you expecting Haylea?'

'They just said this evening. I've got her room ready and my daughter is so excited. Shall I ask Haylea to phone you once she's here? You're bound to be worried about her.'

'Yes, please. That would be good. And Kellie, I think you'll be fine. I've a feeling you're just what Haylea needs right now.'

'Really? Thank you. I'll do my best for her.'

Kellie had sounded gentle and sensitive on the phone and I thought Haylea would find her approachable. Haylea lacked self-confidence and wasn't someone who could easily fit into a group. This was probably one of the reasons she hadn't done well at Waysbury and hadn't been happy at Celia's. Many teenagers thrive in their peer group, but Haylea struggled. Hopefully school would help her form friendship bonds, but for now I thought Kellie and her seven-year-old daughter would provide a good home environment until a specialist carer could be found.

It was eight o'clock when Haylea phoned.

'How's it going?' I asked.

'I think it's OK,' she said hesitantly. 'We've just had dinner.'

'Good. What are you doing now?'

'I'm in the living room with Amelia.'

'Amelia is Kellie's daughter?'

'Yes. Kellie is upstairs unpacking my bag.'

'What time did you get there?' I asked out of interest.

'About six o'clock, I think. Celia had to wait until her husband got home to stay with the boys before she could bring me. I don't think she was very pleased. I said I was sorry for causing her so much trouble. She said it didn't matter as they already had someone else coming tomorrow.' Which I thought was a bit insensitive. She'd made it sound as though fostering was a protection line.

'Don't worry. I'm sure Celia will get over it,' I said. 'I spoke to Kellie on the phone and she sounds very nice. But you will have to tell her if you need anything or if you're worried. She won't know if you don't tell her.'

'I know, she told me that too.'

'Good.'

I heard Amelia say, 'It's your turn, Haylea.'

'Are you playing a game?'

'Yes.'

'I'll let you get on then. Thanks for phoning.'

'Can I call you again if I want?'

'Yes, but try to get some sleep tonight. Kellie is there if you get upset or have a bad dream. I've told her you sometimes have problems sleeping.'

'I'll phone you in the morning.'

'Thanks, love.'

Considering Haylea had only been there a couple of hours, she'd sounded all right. I was pleased she'd had something to eat and was now playing with Amelia. That night I left my phone on anyway, just in case Haylea called, distressed, but she didn't phone, which I took as a good sign. She texted the following morning to say she was awake and going to have breakfast and then a bath. Later that morning she sent a photo of a batch of cupcakes she, Kellie and Amelia had made, which I took as another good sign.

Yummy. They look good x, I texted back.

I received an email from Nia saying she'd set up a meeting with Darcy-May's new adoptive parents for the following Monday. I knew I couldn't take Darcy-May so I phoned Lucy and she was happy to look after her for a few hours while I went to the meeting. Other than making a note in my diary of the meeting, I didn't give it much thought. I was too busy thinking about Haylea and how she was getting on.

Haylea didn't phone that night, but then on Thursday afternoon Kellie phoned. I immediately thought the worst and that something was wrong until she said, 'Haylea has been asking about her other belongings. I think they are still with you?'

'Yes, they are,' I said, relieved. 'Shari will need to make arrangements to get them to Haylea. I'll remind her. She may wait until she moves to her permanent carers.'

'When will that be?'

'I don't know.'

'Have they found someone?' Kellie asked.

'I really don't know. Shari will tell you when there is any news. How is Haylea?'

'She seems all right. She's talking to me and she gets on really well with Amelia. Although Haylea is much older, she seems to like playing children's games. I expect that's because she didn't have much of a childhood herself.'

'Exactly right,' I said. 'You see it so often in fostering when children have been deprived of a childhood. I'm pleased she is settling in.'

'Do you want to talk to her? She's helping Amelia to thread beads to make jewellery.'

'Not if she's busy. Just give her my love.'

'I will.'

Later Haylea sent me a photo of the jewellery she and Amelia had made.

Beautiful x, I replied.

On Saturday Adrian took Paula to the garage to collect her car. They returned a couple of hours later with Paula driving her car behind Adrian in his. He'd wanted to see her home. I immediately went outside to admire the car. She was so proud of it. She spent the next hour cleaning it inside and out, although it was already spotless. Then she took me for a little drive with Darcy-May in her baby seat in the back.

That night as I was getting into bed Haylea phoned and my heart sank.

'What's the matter, love?' I asked, taking the phone out of my bedroom so I wouldn't disturb Darcy-May.

'Can I ask you something, Cathy?' she said in a small, anxious voice.

'Yes, of course, anything.' But I steeled myself for what she was about to say.

'Cathy, I'm alone in my bedroom here and I've been thinking. I don't want to be any more trouble, and I know I can't live with you again, but do you think I can stay with Kellie?'

'Is that what you wanted to ask?'

'Yes.'

'Oh, I see. I don't know. Do you want to stay then?'

'I think so. She's nice and so is Amelia. If I move again, I might get another horrible carer.'

'I don't think Celia could be called horrible, but she wasn't right for you. Have you told Kellie you want to stay?'

'No. I thought I would ask you first.'

This was difficult. 'I think you need to talk to Shari about it. Kellie agreed to have you for a few days. It might be that she was thinking of fostering very young children. I don't know. You will need to ask Shari.'

'Can you tell her?'

'All right, I'll email her.'

'Thank you.'

'But, Haylea, don't get your hopes up. It's possible Shari might not feel it's the best place for you.' Or, I thought but didn't say, Kellie might not agree to have you long term.

CHAPTER TWENTY-SEVEN

SCHOOL

On Monday Paula drove to work in her new car and texted me to say she had arrived and found somewhere to park. She appreciated that as a parent I never stopped worrying about her, even though she was an adult.

I emailed Shari and told her of Haylea's request. Then that afternoon, as I was about to leave the house to take Darcy-May to Lucy so I could attend the adoption meeting, Shari phoned.

'The meeting is off,' she said. 'The couple have pulled out. They've decided to try another course of IVF [in vitro fertilization] instead.'

'But surely that was explored during their assessment to adopt?' I said, exasperated. Applying to adopt is a lengthy process that includes in-depth social-worker assessment and preparation training. They discuss many issues, including the applicant's health and infertility – a primary reason for wanting to adopt. The adopters were also expected to spend time researching adoption and to complete an adoption-journey log. So they'd had plenty of time to consider undergoing more IVF.

'It was explored, and they said they didn't want any more treatment and had decided to adopt instead.

Clearly, they've changed their minds,' Shari said stoically. 'Nia will be in touch when she has identified another couple.'

'Just as well Darcy-May isn't old enough to know,' I said, glancing at her. She was already in her seat, ready to travel in the car.

'Thank you for your email about Haylea wanting to stay at Kellie's,' Shari said, moving on. 'I'm going to visit them on Thursday so I'll discuss that, among other things.'

'Do you want to take the rest of Haylea's belongings with you?' I asked.

'Yes, I could. Just a minute, let me check my diary.'

I smiled at Darcy-May while I waited.

'I can come to you on Wednesday at two o'clock,' Shari said. 'I'll see Darcy-May at the same time.'

'That's fine with me. I'll see you then,' I said, and we ended the call.

I noted Shari's visit in my diary and then telephoned Lucy. I told her the meeting had been cancelled and suggested I still came to see her and Emma.

'Yes, come, that'll be nice,' she said.

I picked up Darcy-May in her car seat and, with the baby bag over my shoulder, left the house and drove to Lucy's flat. When I arrived I made a fuss of Emma while Lucy amused Darcy-May. The weather was good, so we decided to walk to the park. Lucy naturally asked why the meeting had been cancelled and I told her.

'I would adopt her myself if I was younger,' I added.

'I know you would,' she laughed indulgently.

Although fostering is different from adoption, sometimes carers are allowed to adopt the child they are fostering – as I was with Lucy. But babies were placed with young adopters, not someone my age.

We spent a pleasant afternoon in the park and then I returned briefly to Lucy's flat before going home.

On Tuesday I brought down the suitcases from the loft and set about packing the rest of Haylea's belongings. As I worked I talked to Darcy-May, who was watching me from the bed. I'd propped her up with pillows so she couldn't fall off. I always talked to her if we were together and she responded with babbles and lots of arm waving. I wondered if Haylea ever thought about her now she wasn't here. In some ways it was better she'd left before Darcy-May had to go and avoided her final departure from the house, which would surely have affected her on some level. Or would she have remained in denial she'd ever had a baby? It was difficult to know what Haylea was thinking and feeling, as she'd become adept at shutting off her emotions in order to survive the years of abuse. It was something that would hopefully be addressed in therapy.

That evening Kellie telephoned me and again I thought for a moment something was wrong until she said she was thinking of offering Haylea permanency and wanted to know what I thought.

'Haylea has been through so much, I feel right out of my depth,' Kellie admitted. 'But Shari said she'll resume therapy, and Haylea really wants to stay. We've got a meeting here on Thursday and my supervising social worker will come too.'

I sympathized with her dilemma. From what I knew of Kellie she seemed lovely, but it was a huge commitment.

Haylea had only been there a week and faced a difficult time ahead: the court case (assuming her father was prosecuted), starting a new school and coming to terms with everything that had happened to her. Yes, therapy would play a part, but it wouldn't be a complete panacea, not by a long way. At present Haylea was compliant and tended to internalize her feelings, but that could change. How would Kellie feel if Haylea became very angry and disruptive and took it out on her or Amelia? Would she cope?

'See what comes out of the discussion on Thursday,' I suggested. 'Make sure you ask any questions you have and are given all the background information.'

'Shari said she'd email me the Essential Information Forms.'

'Good. But they won't tell you everything, so ask if you have concerns or need more information.'

'Thank you,' she said. 'I want to do what's best for Haylea.'

'I know.'

When Shari visited me on Wednesday I had Haylea's suitcases and bags ready in the hall. We went into the living room where Darcy-May was in her bouncing cradle. I updated Shari on her progress, as was expected, and showed her the Red Book. Satisfied all was well with Darcy-May, Shari then talked about Haylea. I learnt that her father, having broken his bail conditions, would be held on remand in prison until the court case, which was the first week in December.

'So he is definitely going to be prosecuted?' I asked.

'Yes. He's claiming he's innocent,' Shari said. 'But the police are confident they have enough evidence to convict him and two others. They found hundreds of hours of video footage at the houses they searched, some of it going back years and showing Haylea. The older videos are from when she was about eight years old. Her mother was in some too.'

'Her mother participated in the abuse?' I asked, shocked and disgusted.

'It would seem so. The police are trying to trace her.'

I swallowed hard. Bad enough that Haylea's father was a paedophile who had abused his own daughter, but it beggared belief that her mother had too. My stomach curdled. We expect parents to nurture and protect their children unconditionally, not abuse them.

'The police are still trying to identify the other children shown in the videos,' Shari said.

'I pity the police officers who have to view all those videos,' I said, voicing my thoughts. 'You know the niece and nephew of the man who gave those parties?' She nodded. 'Did their parents not suspect anything was wrong?'

'Apparently not. They have told the police that as he was their uncle they saw nothing wrong in him spending time with their children. The children didn't say anything, and we now know they were threatened into silence. Although the parents have admitted the boy had begun bed-wetting and both children had nightmares. They've told their foster carer that their uncle said he could turn into a werewolf who would eat them and their parents if they told. The carer is noting what they say. Which reminds me, I'll be sending a copy of your log notes about Haylea's disclosures to the police. Is it all online?'

'Yes.'

As Shari talked Darcy-May made it clear she'd had enough of sitting in her bouncing cradle, so I took her onto my lap.

'Did Haylea ask you about tracing her siblings?' I asked as Shari finished.

'Yes. We know one of her brothers is in prison, but we don't know the whereabouts of the other brother or her sister. The police want to see them as there is a chance they were abused too. I'll tell Haylea if they're found.'

I nodded solemnly.

Shari ended her visit by looking around the house as she was supposed to. As we returned downstairs and passed the bags and cases in the hall I said, 'There are two more bags of Haylea's clothes in the cupboard under the stairs. Her father bought them for her and she doesn't want them.'

'Get rid of them,' Shari said decisively.

We returned to the living room so Shari could collect her briefcase.

'Do you think Haylea will be allowed to stay with Kellie?' I asked.

'We'll see what tomorrow's meeting brings. They might have fallen out and changed their minds by then.' Which was true.

I sat Darcy-May in her bouncing cradle so I could help Shari load Haylea's bags and cases into her car.

'Have a safe journey tomorrow,' I said, once they were all in.

'Thank you. It's about a three-hour drive.'

* * *

The following day I wondered how the meeting at Kellie's was going and if Haylea would be allowed to stay. Shari didn't need to tell me the outcome as I was no longer fostering Haylea, but shortly after four o'clock Haylea phoned, more excited than I'd heard her in a long while.

'I can stay here,' she said, delighted.

'Good.'

'I'm sorry I couldn't stay with you, but Kellie and Amelia are nice too. Will you come and see me?'

'Yes, once Kellie feels you are settled enough.'

'You're not upset with me for wanting to stay here, are you?'

'No, of course not, love. I'm pleased for you both.'

'I love Kellie and Amelia just like I love you.'

'That is nice.'

'Can I still phone you if I want to?'

'Yes.'

'Kellie wants to speak to you now.'

'OK, love, take care.'

Kellie came on the phone. 'My social worker thought I was up to it,' she said, a note of pride in her voice. 'But there is so much to do. I'll have to register Haylea at my doctor's, find her a new school, get her what she needs and unpack all these bags. Haylea wants to go to the park now, so does Amelia, so I think we'll do that first.'

I could hear the excitement in her voice – that shiny, unbridled enthusiasm of the new foster carer before it became slightly less shiny from the reality of fostering. Not that we ever lose our commitment to fostering, but over time we learn to manage our expectations. To accept we can't always make the difference we had hoped, that decisions in the care system can take longer than we anticipate and are not always the ones we would have made, and there is a lot of form-filling and meetings to attend. But at the heart of it is the child who fuels our passion for fostering.

Now Haylea was settled at Kellie's and I was less preoccupied with worrying about her, I could fully concentrate on Darcy-May. She was six months old now, so I began giving her some weaning food. She looked startled to begin with as the plastic spoon touched her lips and spat out the puréed food. But little by little she began opening her mouth as I offered the spoon and then swallowing. Following current guidelines, I gave her blended vegetables or fruit, and rice mix – a single flavour at a time. Her main nutrition was still coming from the formula milk, so this was to get her used to eating different textures and tastes.

Having only Darcy-May to look after was comparatively easy and I took time to see Lucy and her family, Adrian and Kirsty, and my friends, who often got neglected when there was a lot going on with the children I looked after.

Kellie and Haylea both texted and all seemed to be going well, although a school hadn't been found yet for Haylea. Then halfway through September, when the schools were nearly two weeks into the new term, Haylea phoned late one night. Immediately I thought something must be wrong.

'They've found me a school and I am supposed to start next week,' she said, her voice flat. 'But I don't want to go. I'd rather stay at home with Kellie.'

'You've been out of school a long time,' I said. 'But you'll soon get into the routine. These things are always worse before, then afterwards you wonder what you worried about.'

'All the other kids in the class will be younger than me,' Haylea said. 'Because I've missed so much school I can't go into my proper year.'

'I see.' Students of Haylea's age would normally be in their exam year, but Haylea was nowhere near that level. Not all areas have schools like Turnbridge, and I guessed this was the most appropriate they could find for Haylea in that area. I encouraged her as best I could and also told her to tell Kellie of her worries. She said she had.

The following day I called Kellie just to make sure she was aware how worried Haylea was about starting her new school and what a big step it was for her.

'I know,' Kellie said. 'She's not sleeping or eating well. But she needs to go to school. We were lucky to be offered the place. The schools are full. It's not far away. Only a short bus ride. But it's not just school that's worrying her – it's the court case too.'

'She didn't mention that when she phoned,' I said.

'She can't talk about it, but the police liaison officer phoned and because Haylea's father is pleading not guilty she will have to go to court and be cross-examined by his barrister. It's not until December, so she's got all this time to worry about it. They've told her she will be able to sit behind a screen in court, so she won't have to see her father, but it's still a big ordeal.'

'Yes, it is,' I said. 'Has she resumed therapy yet?'

'No. Shari said she'd chase it up and I have phoned and left messages. I seem to spend hours on the phone trying to find the right person to speak to. I've got Haylea's review and two days' training this week too.'

'But you're still enjoying fostering?' I asked.

'Oh yes. Don't get me wrong, Haylea is lovely, but she does need a lot of attention – more than Amelia.'

'Make sure you spend time with her too,' I said. And I finished by saying if there was anything I could do to help she should let me know.

Nia, from the Family Finding team, telephoned with details of another meeting and another 'excellent match for Darcy-May'. I noted the time and day in my diary and hoped this was the right one. Although I would be very sorry to see Darcy-May leave, for her sake it was important she was settled with her forever family so she could start bonding with them rather than me. The meeting was on Monday, the same day Haylea was due to start school.

That morning I texted Haylea: *Good luck. Thinking of you, Cathy xx*.

But two hours later, as I was preparing the baby bag so I could drop off Darcy-May at Lucy's on my way to the meeting, Kellie phoned.

'Haylea didn't go to school,' she said anxiously.

'No? What happened?

'I took her in my car, but she refused to get out. A member of staff came out and tried talking to her. Haylea has agreed to try again tomorrow, but I have doubts. If she calls you, please tell her she has to go. This is stressing me out.'

'Of course I will, but don't stress. Keep trying, but if Haylea really can't face going to mainstream school then an alternative will have to be found.'

'Like what?'

'She could be home-tutored or attend a school part time. It will depend on what provision there is in your area.'

'And they will let her do that?'

'Yes, if necessary.'

'I wonder if she could attend this school part time, at least to begin with?'

'It's possible. Talk to Haylea and Shari about it and then ask the school.'

'I will, thanks,' she said, brightening a little.

This was something that as an experienced foster carer I knew, but a new carer wouldn't necessarily.

CHAPTER TWENTY-EIGHT

SAM AND NICKY

I arrived at the council offices for the meeting with Darcy-May's prospective adopters five minutes early and made my way up to the room. I knew Joy wouldn't be coming as she had a prior commitment. In my bag was Darcy-May's Life Story Book, a supplementary photograph album and the USB stick containing more photographs and video clips. I knocked on the door of the meeting room and went in. Nia was already seated at the table with two women I guessed to be in their thirties.

'Hi, Cathy,' Nia said brightly. 'This is Nicky and Sam.'

'Hello,' I said, returning their smiles, and sat at the table. 'Nice to meet you.'

When Nia had mentioned the prospective adopters I'd assumed they were a heterosexual couple – wrongly, as it turned out. Of course, same-sex couples can foster and adopt.

'And you,' Nicky said. 'We're so excited.'

'We've been looking forward to this day for ages,' Sam added.

'I can imagine. Adoption is a long process,' I replied.

Both women had medium-length hair and were dressed smart-casual. Their manner was warm and open.

'You must have mixed feelings coming here today,' Nicky said. 'I mean, you've looked after Darcy-May since she was a few days old and this is the first step to parting with her.'

'Yes, that's right,' I agreed, appreciating her sensitivity.

'Can we assure you now that, assuming we're allowed to adopt Darcy-May, we will love and care for her just as you have done?' Sam said.

Immediately I felt my eyes fill.

'We'll send you photographs,' Nicky added. 'And of course you must come to visit us.'

'Thank you,' I said.

The door opened and Shari came in. 'Sorry I'm late,' she said, taking a seat at the table. 'So how far have we got?'

'We've just said hello really,' Nia said.

'Good. As you've all met we'll skip the introductions and get straight to the reason we're here. Cathy, would you like to start by telling Sam and Nicky all about Darcy-May.'

'Yes, of course.' Although we'd had two false starts before, I was already feeling more optimistic.

'This is Darcy-May's Life Story Book,' I said, placing it on the table in front of Sam and Nicky. 'I'll talk while you have a look.'

As they opened the first page they gasped with delight at the photographs of Darcy-May just a few days old. I talked as they turned the pages, commenting on the photos and outlining Darcy-May's progress and development – a week old, two weeks, three weeks, a month and so on, finally coming up to the present day. 'There are plenty of other photographs in this album,' I said, placing that on the table too.

Sam and Nicky pored over this album as Nia and Shari looked at the Life Story Book. 'Very good,' Nia said.

'You've taken so many pictures,' Sam said, glancing up from the album. 'I feel like I'm watching Darcy-May grow.'

Nicky agreed.

'Good, that's the idea, so you haven't missed out on those important first few months. I have more photos, and video clips on this USB,' I said, setting that on the table.

'Perhaps Nicky and Sam could take that home with them to look at later?' Nia suggested.

'Yes, of course.' I handed it to them.

'I'd like us to spend some time answering questions anyone may have,' Nia said.

Sam and Nicky were now going through the photograph album and Life Story Book a second time, their faces a picture of delight and awe. 'Oh my! Look at her there! Beautiful.'

I could see they were both besotted with her and I started to relax.

'Is there anything you would like to ask Cathy?' Shari said, as they came to the end of the albums a second time.

'I don't know. I can't think straight,' Nicky said. 'I feel a bit emotional to be honest.' Her eyes welled as mine had done.

Sam touched her hand tenderly. 'It's OK, love. We've waited a long time for this,' she said.

'Nicky and Sam have been together for ten years,' Nia told me.

'And we've always wanted a family,' Sam said.

'Why go down the adoption route?' I asked.

'You mean, as opposed to conceiving a baby?' Nia asked.

'Yes. It's relatively easy to receive donor sperm. A lot easier than adopting.'

'That's true,' Nicky said. 'But I'm adopted so it seemed the natural choice for us.'

'I see. Do you have any contact with your birth mother?' I asked.

'No. I've never felt the need,' Nicky replied. 'But I am aware that some adopted children do trace their birth parents. That's one of the issues we were asked to think about during our adoption assessment. Darcy-May will grow up knowing she is adopted, like I did. If she decides she does want to trace Haylea when she's older then we'll support her.'

'Assuming Haylea wants to see her,' I pointed out. 'Which is a big if.'

I glanced at Shari and Nia, wondering how much Sam and Nicky knew of Haylea and the circumstances of Darcy-May's birth.

'Yes, Haylea would need to agree, of course,' Nicky said. 'I know Haylea doesn't want anything to do with Darcy-May at present, but she could change her mind in years to come.'

Clearly they had thought this through.

'Sam and Nicky are aware that Darcy-May could be a result of incestuous rape,' Nia said.

'Will you do a DNA test to confirm it?' I asked.

'Only if Sam and Nicky want us to,' Shari said. 'Haylea doesn't want it done.'

'We are not asking for it either,' Sam said. Nicky shook her head in agreement. 'Darcy-May is her own person. She is healthy and if she has inherited any conditions that come to light later then we will seek medical help, just as we would with any child.'

'Will you ever tell Darcy-May she is the result of rape?' I asked.

There was silence for a moment and then Nicky said, 'Probably not. Sam and I have talked about this. Will her life be any better for knowing? I don't think so. If she ever wanted to know all the details surrounding her birth then we would have to be honest. Of course, it's possible that if she did see Haylea in the future then she could find out that way. But we'll deal with that if it arises.'

I was greatly reassured and thought how very different Sam and Nicky were to the other couples who'd applied to adopt Darcy-May. They now asked me about her routine and I included eating and sleeping and that I'd just started her on solids. They asked a few questions and then told me a bit about themselves. They lived in a town about fifty miles away. Both worked and were going to share maternity leave. They showed me some photos on their phones of their home and the area where they lived, which was nice of them. They didn't have to do this; their assessment would have included a report on their home.

The atmosphere in the room was now light, happy and full of hope, as it should be at one of these adoption meetings. My initial concerns had gone. Sam and Nicky came across as compassionate, kind and realistic. They had waited a long time for the opportunity to adopt and I had no doubt they would give Darcy-May the love, care and commitment she so dearly deserved.

Nia and Shari wound up the meeting by outlining the time scale. Because Nicky and Sam were already approved to adopt, this match would now go before the matching panel. They next sat in October. Once the match was approved by them – and there was no reason why it shouldn't be – it would be ratified by their adoption agency, which takes two weeks, then introductions could begin.

'So let's meet again on 2 November with our diaries,' Nia said, checking hers. 'We can plan the introductory meetings and move.'

Sam and Nicky gave little whoops of joy and I smiled.

'Will the introduction period be about two weeks?' I checked. This was usual.

'About that,' Nia said. 'We can slow the pace if necessary.'

We all noted this very important date in our diaries and I put lines through the following two weeks as a reminder to keep them free. Once the introductory phase had begun, it would occupy most of my time until Darcy-May moved in with Nicky and Sam. Shari then asked if there was anything else anyone wanted to say, and closed the meeting.

It had lasted an hour and a half and Nia asked Nicky and Sam to wait behind so she could run through the arrangements for the matching panel. This didn't include me, so I said goodbye and stood. Shari waited behind too, but Nicky and Sam also stood to hug me goodbye. I left the room feeling relieved, but also looking forward to seeing Darcy-May again while I had the chance.

When I arrived at Lucy's it was a bit like a nursery. A friend of hers with a toddler and a baby had dropped by, so there were four little ones. Emma was so pleased to see me. She came straight to me and gave me a big kiss and then sat on my lap, kissing my cheek. I stayed for a cup of tea and then went home where I spent time cuddling and playing with Darcy-May. It was bittersweet and I knew I needed to start preparing myself for the day she would leave.

The following evening Kellie telephoned to say that Haylea hadn't gone to school again and she was trying to arrange a meeting at the school. She sounded frustrated. She said Shari was no longer Haylea's social worker and a new one had been appointed from their local social services. Although this was usual practice, it meant Haylea would have to get used to someone new. Kellie hadn't been able to contact the person yet. I listened sympathetically and gave her what advice I could.

It was Friday before I heard from Kellie again and it seemed a lot had happened during the week for them.

'That school was never going to work, even part time,' Kellie began. 'Haylea is a woman in many respects. She's had a baby and her life experience is so different from her peer group, and they were going to put her in a class of even younger children! So, after much thought, phone calls and discussion, we've decided that Haylea will receive home tuition until next year when she is sixteen and can enrol for a vocational or foundation course at our local college.'

'Well done, that sounds better,' I said. 'And her social worker has agreed?'

'Yes. In the meantime, I'll teach Haylea as best I can using online lessons. I've made it clear to Haylea she needs to learn and not spend all her days baking and watching television.'

'Good for you. I think it's the best solution.'

'So do I. They don't tell you things like this in the induction programme for fostering. It's been a sharp learning curve for me.'

'To be honest, you never stop learning in fostering.'

Kellie then put Haylea on the phone and she sounded happy too. 'I don't have to go to school,' she said.

'No, but you do have to continue your education at home.'

'I know.'

We chatted for a while longer and then said goodbye. I completely agreed with Kellie. Haylea would have really struggled in mainstream school, even with support and a reduced timetable. It would have been an additional stress for them both, and Haylea's mental health came first. She would catch up with her education in time.

Two days later Joy telephoned to ask if I could take another child. I said I'd rather not until after Darcy-May had left in November, as it would be difficult once the introductions started. She appreciated my reasons and said she would make a note on their system that I wasn't available at present unless it was an emergency placement.

September slipped into October. The long, hot summer abruptly ended and autumn arrived in earnest. A strong wind blew from the north and trees began to shed their leaves. I still took Darcy-May out each day, and I spent time with Lucy and Emma during the week and saw Paula and Adrian at weekends. Darcy-May's next review had been scheduled for the end of October, but it was decided to postpone it until after she'd moved in with her parents. Technically Darcy-May would still be in care until the adoption order was made by the Family Court.

Haylea and Kellie phoned a few times and all seemed to be going well, although I knew from Kellie that Haylea was very worried about the court case. Kellie said if she tried to talk to her about it, she just zoned out and fell silent. They had met the new social worker and Haylea had started therapy again at CAMHS (Child and Adolescent Mental Health Services) in their area.

On 2 November I attended the meeting to plan the introduction and move of Darcy-May to her parents. Nicky, Sam, Shari, Nia and Joy were present. Darcy-May was with Lucy again. I took some recent photos of her with me. Even in a month they could see she had grown. I showed Sam and Nicky her Red Book, which I would pass to them at the end of the move, together with her Life Story Book and photos. They already had a copy of her medical assessment.

Nia led the meeting and it was decided that the first week of introductions – starting the following day – would take place at my house with a two-hour visit. The second week, culminating in the move, would be at their home. During the two weeks Sam and Nicky would be gradually taking over the care of Darcy-May so that when I left her with them for the last time it wasn't such a big step for her or them. Shari mentioned that Haylea had been offered a goodbye contact with Darcy-May, but had refused. I wasn't surprised. Neither did she want any post-adoption updates or contact.

When I collected Darcy-May from Lucy she asked how the meeting had gone and I said very well. She, like me, felt mixed emotions: that although Sam and Nicky were lovely and right for Darcy-May, we would all miss her dreadfully. This would be the last time Lucy looked after Darcy-May and possibly saw her, so she said a fond goodbye and little Emma gave her a big kiss on the cheek.

I told Paula about the meeting over dinner. She would miss Darcy-May as much as me, as she'd lived with her all this time and helped in her care. That evening she spent a lot of time with Darcy-May, and bathed her and got her ready for bed. I heard her talking to her. 'You are going to meet your new mummies tomorrow.'

Darcy-May chuckled happily.

CHAPTER TWENTY-NINE

ANOTHER CHILD?

Nicky and Sam were both in tears as they held their daughter for the first time, which of course set me off. I passed around the box of tissues and we laughed as we dried our eyes.

'Whatever will Darcy-May think of us?' Nicky said.

'Not much,' Sam agreed.

'She will think she is very lucky,' I said, which set them both off again.

It was a very emotional meeting and had I needed any proof that they were good people who would love and cherish Darcy-May, I had it during the introductions.

On their first visit I stayed in the living room with them as they took turns holding Darcy-May and then feeding her. I talked a lot about Darcy-May, passing on information, and they asked questions about her care, routine, likes and dislikes. Even at seven months, she had preferences. When she needed a clean nappy I showed them upstairs to my room where everything they needed was kept and then stood back to let them change her. They had some experience of babies as Sam had two nieces and some of their friends had children.

'At her age Darcy-May could go in her own bedroom with a baby monitor,' I said. 'But I thought she may as well stay here for now to avoid the disruption.'

'We've put her cot in with us,' Nicky said. 'But her room is ready. Once she's settled, we can see about moving her. All we need to buy are some more clothes. We didn't get too many as she's growing so fast and friends have given us lots too.'

The two hours flew by and it was soon time for Nicky and Sam to leave. They would return tomorrow. They took some photographs of Darcy-May on their phones before they left to send to family and friends.

The next day followed a similar pattern and included them spoon-feeding Darcy-May her lunch, and I left them alone for longer. The next day they took her out in the stroller and then returned to spend the whole afternoon with her.

So the week progressed, building their contact with Darcy-May as mine reduced. By the end of the first week Nicky and Sam were with me for most of the day, caring for Darcy-May as I busied myself in another room or popped out to the shops. I made us lunch and dinner and they met Paula, then they bathed Darcy-May and settled her in her cot before leaving.

During the week Nia and Shari phoned us all to see how the introductions were going and if we were on course for next week, where they would continue at their house. We had one day free at the weekend to give us all a break, and then I drove Darcy-May to what would shortly be her new home. It was a modern terraced house with a neat front garden. A box of early-years toys was in their living room, and Darcy-May recognized them both. But despite our best efforts, these surroundings were new for Darcy-May and she was unsettled and clingy on the first visit. I took her home after two hours as arranged, and then returned the next day for longer, and the next. Her new home gradually became more familiar. I was present, but it was Sam and Nicky who looked after her. I met Sam's parents and also a friend who stopped by. Then I left Darcy-May there for a few hours and explored the neighbouring town. She was now taking her afternoon nap in her cot in their bedroom with the soft toys and blanket from my house, which would smell and feel familiar to her. Those would stay with her when she left me.

When moving an older child to permanency it's usual for them to stay at least one, if not two, nights at their new home before the move, returning to the carers in between, but that could be confusing for a baby. So, in line with the timetable, at the end of the second week Darcy-May stayed overnight and I went home and then returned the next day so she could see me. She'd been restless during the night, but that was only to be expected, and Sam and Nicky had dealt with it by giving her a bottle, which had got her back to sleep. They admitted that they'd stayed awake most of the night listening out for her. It was as new for them as it was for her.

We had two more overnights and then it was time for me to make the last trip. Paula had already had to say goodbye to Darcy-May and wished me luck before she left for work. I set off soon after with the rest of Darcy-May's belongings, including the Red Book and details of her savings account.

Of course I'd known this day would come and I was happy for all three of them, but that didn't make it any easier. Sam and Nicky were subdued too as they greeted me, empathizing with my feelings. They made me a coffee and then played with Darcy-May while I drank it. She was relaxed in their company now and went to them rather than me, so the introductory period had been a success.

I stayed for about an hour and then stood to leave. I said that rather than bring her to the front door, it was probably better if I said my goodbyes in the living room. I put on a brave face as I held and cuddled her, as I didn't want to upset her, but once I'd turned away the tears slipped down my cheeks. I hurried to their front door. Sam came after me, but I waved her away. 'I'll be OK,' I said, and went out, closing the door behind me.

I got into my car and then drove around the corner to compose myself before the drive home. A minute later my phone bleeped with a text message.

Thank you so much for everything. See you soon. Love Sam, Nicky and DM xxx.

They'd started calling her DM, which I thought was rather nice. Even so, I began the drive home with a heavy heart. I passed shops already decorated for Christmas and was reminded that I needed to get going with my Christmas shopping. We were approaching the end of November and I was behind this year with my shopping. Normally I'd made a start by now, but I'd been very busy with Darcy-May and also, if I'm honest, I was struggling as this would be our first Christmas without my mother. I knew I had to deal with it.

Once home, I kept busy. I stripped the cot and put it in

the spare bedroom together with the changing mat and other baby equipment. I cleared up the living room, wrote my log notes on Darcy-May for the last time and emailed Nia, Shari and Joy to say the move had gone well. I then set about preparing dinner for when Paula came home, thinking about Darcy-May and Haylea. It had been a strange year of fostering – with Darcy-May and then her mother. Unusual, and not without its challenges, but that's the nature of fostering, and each child's story is different. You do what you can to help and hope for the best.

Two days before the court case Haylea texted to say she didn't have to go to court but didn't say why. Then Kellie phoned and explained. Haylea's father had changed his plea to guilty – not to save Haylea having to go to court, but because it would reduce his sentence. The other two men also charged were pleading guilty. Kellie said there was so much evidence they were sure to be convicted. She was pleased, as I was. Haylea had been saved the ordeal of going to court, and she said she'd let me know the outcome of the court case.

The next day Joy telephoned.

'Well done. The move went well then,' she said, having read my email about Darcy-May.

'Yes.'

She took a breath and I could guess what was coming next – details of another child. I wasn't wrong. 'We're going to court next week to try to remove a two-year-old as a result of neglect. If the care order is granted, will you be able to take him?'

'Yes.'

303

'Thank you. I'll pass on your details to his social worker.'

'OK.'

So he could be with us for Christmas, I thought. I'd need to add presents for him to my list.

CHAPTER THIRTY

REUNIONS

I began Christmas shopping in earnest, and the first Sunday in December Paula and I put up the decorations. On Monday I heard from Joy that the judge in the court case for the two-year-old the social services wanted to bring into care had adjourned the hearing for a week, as she was missing a report. He would be staying with his mother for now.

Kellie phoned and told me Haylea's father and the two other men on trial had all been found guilty. Despite a reduction in their sentences for pleading guilty, Haylea's father was given ten years and the other two men – one of whom was the owner of the house where the 'parties' had been held – eight years each. Kellie and Haylea were relieved, as I was. While no sentence was long enough for the damage they'd done to Haylea and the other children, at least they couldn't do any more harm and were being punished. When they were released they would be placed on the sex offenders' register and monitored by the police. Kellie said the investigation into the paedophile ring was still ongoing so there was a chance others could be prosecuted too – thanks to Haylea's courage in speaking out. Although

Haylea's father and brother had previous criminal records, they were for robbery and assault. There had been nothing to suggest her father had been sexually abusing Haylea and other children.

Kellie suggested that I might like to visit them before my next child arrived, which seemed a good idea. As it was a three-hour car journey, she said I could stay the night with them. I accepted and drove there the following week with their Christmas presents. I met Amelia, Kellie's seven-year-old daughter, for the first time. A lovely child – confident, mature and respectful. They were all pleased to see me, as I was them. It was clear straight away that Haylea had bonded with her new family; she and Amelia were like sisters.

As Kellie and I talked I learnt that Haylea's birth sister had been found. The girls had spoken on the phone and also video-chatted online so they could see each other. She too had been abused by their father, although not to the extent Haylea had as she'd run away from home. She felt bad now for leaving Haylea to fend for herself and had made a statement to the police giving details of what had happened to her. She and Haylea were planning to meet at some point. The brother who wasn't in prison had also been traced and was living abroad. Haylea's mother, thought to have taken part in some of the abuse, hadn't been found.

I spent a lovely day with them and felt as though I was on holiday, with my meals made and cups of tea brought to me. That night Amelia kindly gave up her bed so I could have it and she slept with her mother. Out of habit I found myself listening out for Haylea, although there was no need now. She was sleeping better, and if she did wake and needed reassuring, it would be Kellie who went to her.

The following morning they made me breakfast and I left soon after, thanking them and wishing them a merry Christmas. I hoped to see them again, but that would largely depend on Haylea. She was clearly settled with Kellie and didn't really need me any more.

At the weekend, while I was still child-free, I arranged to visit Nicky and Sam. They had sent photos of Darcy-May to my phone, which I'd shared with Paula, Lucy and Adrian. Paula came with me, slightly apprehensive and wondering how she would feel seeing Darcy-May again, and if Darcy-May would be upset. However, a month is a long time in a baby's life. When we first arrived she looked at us slightly oddly and then got on with what she was doing – playing with some stacking beakers. It was obvious she had little or no memory of us and was definitely Sam and Nicky's daughter.

They made us feel very welcome and thanked us for the presents I put under their Christmas tree. It would be Darcy-May's first Christmas and the house was festooned with banners and balloons announcing 'Our Baby's First Christmas'. She'd grown since we'd last seen her and was crawling more confidently, pulling herself up by holding onto the furniture or her mothers' legs. She was going through a phase of putting objects in her mouth and Nicky said she was teething. Sam made us hot drinks and served homemade sweet mince pies with flaky pastry, just like my mother used to make. As we talked, they said that when DM was about eighteen months old they would start the adoption process again so that she would have a brother or sister. They asked how Haylea was, which was nice, and having just seen her I could reassure them she was doing well.

We stayed for two hours, during which time Darcy-May was the centre of attention, and then, wishing them a merry Christmas, we kissed Darcy-May goodbye and left.

'I'm glad I came,' Paula said as we got into the car. 'It was reassuring to see her happy and settled. They will have a great Christmas.'

'Yes, and so will we.'

I was looking forward to Christmas now. My family and I would all be together for Christmas day, and Emma was caught up in the excitement. Last Christmas she'd been a baby and had spent most of it on my mother's lap. What a lovely memory that was.

I was still on standby to foster the two-year-old boy Joy had mentioned, but the closer it got to Christmas the more I hoped – indeed, assumed – he would be able to stay with his family, at least for Christmas.

It wasn't to be. Two days before Christmas Joy phoned.

'The judge has granted the care order. His social worker is collecting him from home now and should be with you later today.'

'That poor family. Couldn't he have stayed for Christmas?' I asked.

'No. The mother left him alone all last night while she was out partying.'

I tell their story and continue our fostering journey into the pandemic in my next book. I hope you will join us again. For an update on the children in my fostering memoirs, please visit www.cathyglass.co.uk. Thank you. Take care and God bless. xxx

SUGGESTED TOPICS FOR READING-GROUP DISCUSSION

What is your first impression of Haylea? How does she change during the book? Discuss why she struggles to fit in with her peer group.

Do you think it was the right decision to place Haylea with Cathy?

How much sympathy do you have for Jessica and Andrew's decision not to adopt?

As well as telling Haylea's story, Cathy continues the story of her own family. Why do you think this is important and popular with readers?

Do you think Haylea will ever want to see Darcy-May? If so, in what circumstances might this happen?

How is disclosing abuse and being able to tell the police cathartic?

Discuss Nicky and Sam's approach to adoption and telling Darcy-May of her past.

The book ends as a new child is about to arrive, two days before Christmas. How will Cathy and her family adapt their Christmas and do the best for him?

Cathy Glass

————

One remarkable woman, more
than **150** foster children cared for.

Cathy Glass has been a foster carer for
twenty-five years, during which time she has
looked after more than 150 children, as well
as raising three children of her own. She was
awarded a degree in education and psychology
as a mature student, and writes under a
pseudonym. To find out more about Cathy
and her story visit **www.cathyglass.co.uk**.

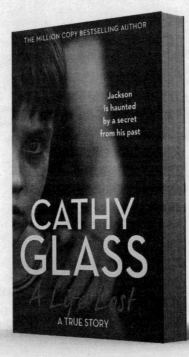

THE MILLION COPY BESTSELLING AUTHOR

Jackson
is haunted
by a secret
from his past

CATHY
GLASS

A True Story

A Lost Life

Jackson is aggressive, confrontational and often volatile

Then, in a dramatic turn of events, the true reason for Jackson's behaviour comes to light . . .

A Terrible Secret

Tilly is so frightened of her stepfather, Dave, that she asks to go into foster care

The more Cathy learns about Dave's behaviour, the more worried she becomes …

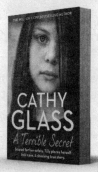

Too Scared to Tell

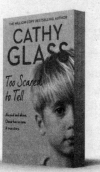

Oskar has been arriving at school hungry, unkempt and bruised. His mother has gone abroad and left him in the care of 'friends'

As the weeks pass, Cathy's concerns deepen. Oskar is clearly frightened of someone – but who? And why?

Innocent

Siblings Molly and Kit arrive at Cathy's frightened, injured and ill

The parents say they are not to blame. Could the social services have got it wrong?

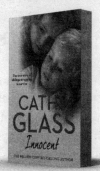

Finding Stevie

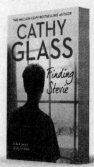

Fourteen-year-old Stevie is exploring his gender identity

Like many young people, he spends time online, but Cathy is shocked when she learns his terrible secret.

Where Has Mummy Gone?

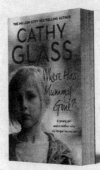

When Melody is taken into care, she fears her mother won't cope alone

It is only when Melody's mother vanishes that what has really been going on at home comes to light.

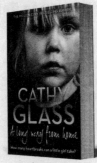

A Long Way from Home

Abandoned in an orphanage, Anna's future looks bleak until she is adopted

Anna's new parents love her, so why does she end up in foster care?

Cruel to be Kind

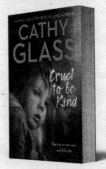

Max is shockingly overweight and struggles to make friends

Cathy faces a challenge to help this unhappy boy.

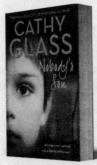

Nobody's Son

Born in prison and brought up in care, Alex has only ever known rejection

He is longing for a family of his own, but again the system fails him.

Can I Let You Go?

Faye is 24, pregnant and has learning difficulties as a result of her mother's alcoholism

Can Cathy help Faye learn enough to parent her child?

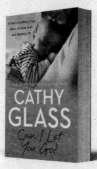

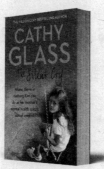

The Silent Cry

A mother battling depression. A family in denial

Cathy is desperate to help before something terrible happens.

Girl Alone

An angry, traumatized young girl on a path to self-destruction

Can Cathy discover the truth behind Joss's dangerous behaviour before it's too late?

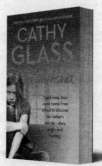

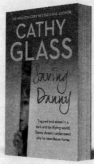

Saving Danny

Danny's parents can no longer cope with his challenging behaviour

Calling on all her expertise, Cathy discovers a frightened little boy who just wants to be loved.

The Child Bride

A girl blamed and abused for dishonouring her community

Cathy discovers the devastating truth.

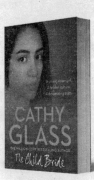

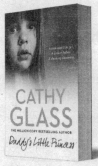

Daddy's Little Princess

A sweet-natured girl with a complicated past

Cathy picks up the pieces after events take a dramatic turn.

Will You Love Me?

A broken child desperate for a loving home

The true story of Cathy's adopted daughter Lucy.

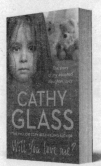

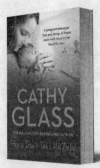

Please Don't Take My Baby

Seventeen-year-old Jade is pregnant, homeless and alone

Cathy has room in her heart for two.

Another Forgotten Child

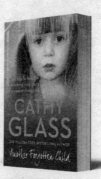

Eight-year-old Aimee was on the child-protection register at birth

Cathy is determined to give her the happy home she deserves.

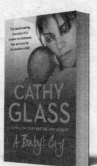

A Baby's Cry

A newborn, only hours old, taken into care

Cathy protects tiny Harrison from the potentially fatal secrets that surround his existence.

The Night the Angels Came

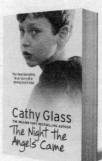

A little boy on the brink of bereavement

Cathy and her family make sure Michael is never alone.

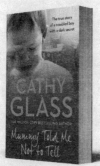

Mummy Told Me Not to Tell

A troubled boy sworn to secrecy

After his dark past has been revealed, Cathy helps Reece to rebuild his life.

I Miss Mummy

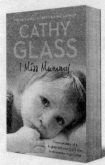

Four-year-old Alice doesn't understand why she's in care

Cathy fights for her to have the happy home she deserves.

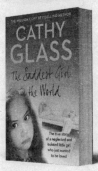

The Saddest Girl in the World

A haunted child who refuses to speak

Do Donna's scars run too deep for Cathy to help?

Cut

Dawn is desperate to be loved

Abused and abandoned, this vulnerable child pushes Cathy and her family to their limits.

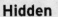

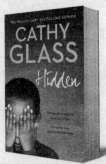

Hidden

The boy with no past

Can Cathy help Tayo to feel like he belongs again?

Damaged

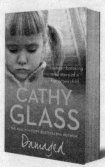

A forgotten child

Cathy is Jodie's last hope. For the first time, this abused young girl has found someone she can trust.

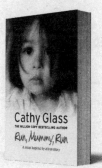

Run, Mummy, Run

The gripping story of a woman caught in a horrific cycle of abuse, and the desperate measures she must take to escape.

My Dad's a Policeman

The dramatic short story about a young boy's desperate bid to keep his family together.

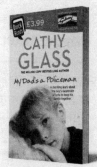

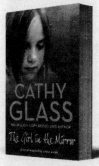

The Girl in the Mirror

Trying to piece together her past, Mandy uncovers a dreadful family secret that has been blanked from her memory for years.

About Writing
and How to Publish

A clear, concise practical
guide on writing and the best
ways to get published.

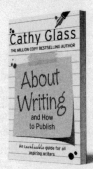

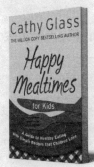

Happy Mealtimes
for Kids

A guide to healthy eating
with simple recipes that
children love.

Happy Adults

A practical guide to achieving lasting
happiness, contentment and success.
The essential manual for getting
the best out of life.

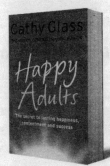

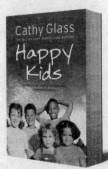

Happy Kids

A clear and concise guide to
raising confident, well-behaved
and happy children.

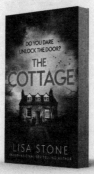
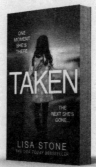

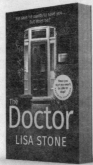

THE DOCTOR

How much do you know about
the couple next door?

STALKER

Security cameras are there to
keep us safe. Aren't they?

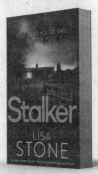

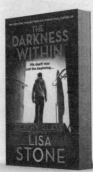

THE DARKNESS
WITHIN

You know your son better than
anyone. Don't you?

Be amazed
Be moved
Be inspired

Follow Cathy:

⊕ /cathy.glass.180

🐦 @CathyGlassUK

www.cathyglass.co.uk

Cathy loves to hear from readers and reads
and replies to posts, but she asks that no plot
spoilers are posted, please. We're sure
you appreciate why.

MOVING
Memoirs

Stories of hope, courage and
the power of love . . .

Sign up to the Moving Memoirs email and you'll
be the first to hear about new books, discounts,
and get sneak previews from your
favourite authors!

Sign up at

www.moving-memoirs.com